*Biofeedback* FOR THE BRAIN

## DATE DUE

| | | | |
|---|---|---|---|
| SEP 27 2011 | | | |
| 12/2/13 ILL | | | |
| OCT 0 6 2022 | | | |
| | | | |
| | | | |
| | | | |
| | | | |
| | | | |
| | | | |
| | | | |
| | | | |
| | | | |
| | | | |
| | | | |
| | | | |
| | | | |

Demco, Inc. 38-293

# Biofeedback

# FOR THE BRAIN

How Neurotherapy

Effectively Treats

Depression,

ADHD, Autism,

and More

*Paul G. Swingle, Ph.D.*

RUTGERS UNIVERSITY PRESS

NEW BRUNSWICK, NEW JERSEY, AND LONDON

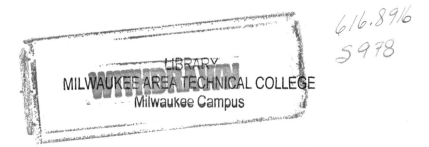

First paperback printing, 2010

Library of Congress Cataloging-in-Publication Data

Swingle, Paul G.

Biofeedback for the brain : how neurotherapy effectively treats depression, ADHD, autism, and more /
Paul G. Swingle.

p. cm.

Includes bibliographical references and index.

ISBN 978-0-8135-4287-4 (hardcover : alk. paper)

ISBN 978-0-8135-4779-4 (pbk. : alk. paper)

1. Biofeedback training.    2. Brain—Diseases—
Treatment.    I. Title.

RC489.B53S95 2008

616.89'16—dc22                          2007024979

A British Cataloging-in-Publication record for this
book is available from the British Library.

Text design by Adam B. Bohannon

Visit our Web site:

http://rutgerspress.rutgers.edu

Manufactured in
the United States of America

# CONTENTS

# FIGURES AND TABLES

*Biofeedback* FOR THE BRAIN

# Introduction: "It's All in Your Head"

In his book *A Symphony in the Brain,* journalist Jim Robbins wonders why a field with such enormous promise as neurotherapy is still not well known. It has been practiced by therapists for almost four decades. Numerous studies have shown that it can treat serious mental conditions. Further, neurotherapy has been shown to be effective for conditions that many people feel they must endure for the rest of their lives. Neurotherapy treats these debilitating conditions without drugs or side effects, and it performs, in Robbins's words, "what most of us have been conditioned to think of as miracles."[1] In a similar vein, Frank Duffy, pediatric neurologist at Harvard Medical School, states that neurotherapy "is a field to be taken seriously by all."[2]

As a well-known expert with thirty years of experience in the field, I have written this book to tell readers what neurotherapy is, how it works, and how it can help you, a loved one, or, if you are a health care professional, your clients and patients. Neurotherapy can treat many conditions, including attention deficit disorder (ADD), depression, anxiety disorders, sleep problems, brain damage from head injuries, epilepsy, and alcoholism and other addictions. It has been shown to be helpful even for conditions often considered untreatable beyond maintenance and sedation, such as autism and psychosis. Neurotherapy treats these conditions by changing the way the brain functions. Although this seems at first to be a daunting notion, it is quite simple and logical. Brain functions that are not efficient are "exercised" to make them more efficient. Similar to physical exercise to strengthen specific muscles in the body, neurotherapy increases the efficiency of specific brain functions. It safely corrects many inefficiencies in the brain that cause problems.

*Neurotherapy* refers to several different, but related, methods for modifying brainwave activity. *Neurofeedback,* also known as brainwave biofeedback, is the fundamental form of neurotherapy. Simply stated, neurofeedback provides clients with direct feedback about the state of particular brainwave activity. The feedback can be sound or visual images on a computer monitor or stimulation of the skin (for example, vibration) that lets the client know about brainwave activity that the client cannot feel. Clients make use of the feedback to learn how to control their brainwave activity. For example, a client may hear a tone when the brain is functioning in a more efficient manner than before. The client uses that information to learn how to increase the time the brain is functioning efficiently. As the brain functioning becomes increasingly efficient, the symptoms associated with the inefficient functioning start to improve. This process is similar to a client doing physical exercise for a specific problem such as poor hand-grip strength. As the client does the exercise, the muscle strengthens and the grip becomes increasingly strong. Several different neurotherapeutic methods used to modify brainwave functioning are discussed throughout this book. However, brainwave biofeedback remains the most important form of neurotherapy for the vast majority of the disorders that neurotherapists treat.

**NEUROFEEDBACK**
Neurofeedback, also called brainwave biofeedback, is a self-regulatory treatment to normalize and optimize brain functioning. Brainwave activity is monitored, electronically, from electrodes placed on the scalp. The neurotherapist sets conditions that let the client know when brainwave activity is moving in the desired direction. Thus, for example, the client may hear a tone when the brain is producing brainwaves that are related to calming. Or a child might see a bug move more quickly on the computer monitor when brainwaves related to poor focus become weaker. These biofeedback procedures move the brain toward efficient functioning.

Brain functioning has begun to arouse the interest of the media. Many major publications, such as the *National Geographic,* have published major articles on the brain. Specifically, the concept of changing brain functioning to modify behavior has been getting media coverage. For example, in the 2005 inaugural issue of *Scientific American*'s journal *Mind,* neurotherapy was said to be the "latest leap" for treating attention deficit hyperactivity disorders (ADHD). The *Wall Street Journal* published an article on neurofeedback training to give athletes the mental edge, citing as one example neurofeedback training done with soccer players on the winning Italian World Cup team in 2006. In this case, the increased efficiency of the players' brains was reflected in their improved athletic performance.[3] Similarly, neurotherapy can correct or improve the anomalies in brain functioning that are responsible for many disorders. If a person suffers from poor sleep, for example, the functioning of the area of the brain responsible for sleep is enhanced, and the quality of the person's sleep is improved.

In 1968, in the journal *Physiology and Behavior,* M. Barry Sterman, a psychologist at the University of California, Los Angeles School of Medicine, published the results of his experiments training cats to control their own brainwaves.[4] Later, in 1972, Sterman published the first scientific paper about using brainwave feedback to suppress seizures in a twenty-three-year-old woman.[5] These early studies at Sterman's laboratories demonstrated that brain activity can be modified with behavioral methods.

Although perhaps surprising, self-regulation of brain activity has been practiced for thousands of years in meditation, yoga, and the martial arts. Elmer Green, at the Menninger Clinic in Topeka, Kansas, observed that people practiced in meditation produced high-amplitude slow-frequency brain signals when in profoundly relaxed states. Green further reported on the use of brainwave biofeedback to increase slow-frequency brainwave amplitudes to enhance hypnotic relaxed states.[6] Like yogis for thousands of years, twentieth-century practitioners and scientists tapped into the power of the mind to influence its own activity, a practice that leads to states of enhanced mental clarity and relaxation. Eugene Peniston at the Fort Lyons, Colorado, Veterans Administration Hospital applied these same biofeedback techniques in the first controlled scientific study of the brainwave treatment of alcoholism.[7] Peniston found that genetically predisposed alcoholics were deficient in slow-frequency brainwave amplitudes relative to fast-frequency amplitudes in the back of the brain. Using a brainwave biofeedback treatment similar to that

used by Green at the Menninger, Peniston increased the relative amplitude of the slow brainwaves with marked success in the treatment of
institutionalized alcoholics.

So the field of neurotherapy is not new. What is new and exciting is
the rapidly developing use of these techniques in the treatment of many
disorders and for optimizing performance. Neurotherapists gently and
safely assist their clients to gain control over their brainwave activity and
then to self-regulate that activity into increasingly efficient functioning.
Brainwave biofeedback allows clients to gain control over their brain
activity by providing immediate feedback on brainwave changes. Clients
learn to gain control by focusing on the feedback and by experimenting to achieve improved mental and physical states, just as the yogis of
old did. As a result, the feedback signals stay in the positive range. However, brainwave biofeedback can accomplish in a matter of weeks the
results that the yogis might accomplish in ten or more years. Neurotherapy is fast becoming a primary-care choice for many patients who
want safe and natural methods for dealing with medical and psychological disorders. Rather than take a medication, clients gain control over
brain functioning to correct the source of the problem. Because of the
precise brainwave evaluations done prior to treatment, the exact location
and nature of the neurological predispositions are isolated. The brainwave biofeedback focuses specifically and precisely on the problematic
brain locations and assists clients to control and correct the brainwave
functioning.

Medical and psychological authorities have scientifically validated
these procedures. The equipment used is registered with the Federal
Drug Administration (FDA) and complies with the FDA's regulations
for medical devices. Duffy, pediatric neurologist and professor at
Harvard Medical School, states in the medical journal *Clinical EEG,* "The
literature, which lacks any negative study of substance, suggests that
EEG [electroencephalogram] biofeedback therapy should play a major
therapeutic role in many difficult areas. In my opinion, if any medication
had demonstrated such a wide spectrum of efficiency it would be
universally accepted and widely used."[8] In short, brainwave biofeedback
is a safe and effective treatment for a wide variety of disorders.

Many clients tell me that after making the rounds of health care
providers who have not been able to help, they end up in a psychiatrist's

office. Many of these clients, struggling with neurological and psychological symptoms, find that our health care system typically blames the client for not getting better; hence, the referral to the psychologist or psychiatrist. The client soon understands that the referring physician believes that the client's problems are not valid in a medical sense but are a function of the client's mental condition. My response to clients who have been told, "It's all in your head," is "Of course, where else would it be?" The client is experiencing symptoms because the brain is not functioning efficiently. Thus, neurotherapy treats the problem where it resides—in the client's head. Clients who find a well-trained, certified, and licensed neurotherapy provider are on their way to a safe, natural, data-guided treatment that corrects problems rather than sedates them. (For advice about selecting a neurotherapist, see the Appendix.)

**FREQUENTLY ASKED QUESTION**

Q: My eight-year-old's teacher said she needs Ritalin. I don't agree. What should I do?

A: I would thank the teacher for her concern, tell her you are addressing the problem using nonmedication approaches, and take your daughter to a neurotherapist for assessment and, if necessary, for treatment. Also, ask the teacher to inform you of your daughter's progress in school.

On the first visit, a neurotherapist usually does a brainwave assessment. This assessment is an advanced form of the EEG, which measures brainwaves. The therapist measures the brain's activity at several locations on the head. The EEG uses miniature electrodes that are attached to each ear and some on the head. The client feels nothing because the EEG is for measurement only. The client may be asked to open and close the eyes and to read or count; the client may also be exposed to some form of stimulation such as sounds or lights to determine the brain's reaction to these conditions. After the EEG data are obtained, the neurotherapist analyzes the results and often can immediately provide the client with a detailed assessment of the symptoms. As we will review in detail throughout this book, the brain "tells us everything" in the sense of identifying symptoms based exclusively on the brainwave data. To clients' surprise, the neurotherapist can often tell them why they have come for treatment without any additional information about their condition. After reviewing the symptoms, the neurotherapist then shows the client precisely where in the brain the EEG biofeedback will be done to correct the brainwave activity and thereby correct the symptoms.

Usually, when I tell a family that their child has one of several forms of ADHD that can be treated with brainwave biofeedback, both the parents and the child give a profound sigh of relief. In one case, the father called me a few days after the initial office visit and told me that my diagnosing his son as having ADHD was the "best Christmas present my family had ever received!" He went on to say that the whole family was emotionally reunited and joyous. The good news was that the child, and the family, received definitive information on the cause of the child's difficulties. He was not stupid or lazy. He was not worthless or unlovable. He simply had an inefficiency in the way his brainwaves functioned. And I gave the family more good news when I told them how the ADHD symptoms could be improved, permanently, without drugs.

Neurotherapy has emerged since the mid-1970s as a safe procedure that permits rapid, accurate diagnoses and treatment of many common disorders. Practitioners of neurotherapy do not use surgery on the brain to learn its secrets. The electrical currents inside the head can be measured from the outside. The treatment I provide was once called "bloodless brain surgery" by a patient of mine who experienced a marked reduction in symptoms that had remained unchanged after many years of both conventional medical and alternative treatments.

When clients tell me about their problems, my job is not to label the problem but rather to discover the neurological basis for it. Children may have problems in school for any number of reasons. Simply labeling the behavior as ADHD is not going to help the child because ADHD can have multiple causes. Indeed, it might be a food allergy or a thyroid problem rather than a neurologically based problem. In the short term, drugs such as Ritalin and some newer forms of central-nervous-system stimulants may temporarily improve attention and reduce hyperactivity, but they are less effective than neurotherapy in improving academic and social performance. In addition, growing evidence shows the dangers of having children take drugs for a long time. Controlled scientific studies have compared the effects of Ritalin and other stimulants with the effects of brainwave biofeedback. Both approaches can result in significant improvements in behavior and attention, but if the drug is stopped, the problems return, whereas children treated with brainwave biofeedback sustain their gains. For example, Vincent Monastra, professor of psychology at the State University of New York at Binghamton, and his colleagues studied one hundred children between the ages of six and nineteen diagnosed with ADHD. Half the children received neurofeedback in addition to medication, while the other half received only stimulant medication. All the children received some educational support, and parents also received some parenting advice. Only the group receiving the neurofeedback sustained their improvement when the stimulant drug was withdrawn.[9]

Other controlled scientific studies have likewise shown that neurofeedback can permanently improve deficiencies in attention. The safe and lasting neurofeedback intervention, though more time consuming, is a much healthier choice than medication. Relying on stimulants to treat the disorder does nothing to lessen the chronic nature of ADHD and other neurobehavioral conditions. Long-term use of stimulant medications also exposes the child, and later the adult, to serious health risks. A wide array of psychological and neurological disorders can affect a person's ability to concentrate. Stress, pain, depression, anxiety, sleep disturbance, addictions, diet and food sensitivities, hormone disturbances, fatigue, and so on all affect our ability to be aware of our environment. Our ability to focus and comprehend is central to every facet of our existence. In order to enjoy the richness of life, we should not have to spend years taking drugs such as Ritalin or Prozac.

Brainwave-modification treatment is not complicated. Brainwaves are electrical signals from the brain that can be measured from the surface of the skull. Also known as EEG, these brainwaves indicate how the brain is functioning. As discussed previously, the neurotherapist uses the EEG to determine the exact nature of the client's symptoms. Specific brainwave patterns are associated with specific physical and mental states. For example, several brainwave patterns are associated with a predisposition to depression. In addition, certain brainwave frequencies (cycles per second), such as from 8 to 12 cycles per second (alpha), are identified by letters of the Greek alphabet based on when they were identified. (Alpha, for example, was the first to be identified.) When you are in deep sleep, your brain produces slow activity, known as delta waves. When you drift off, as just before sleep, the brain produces theta waves. Theta waves are a bit faster in frequency than delta waves but are still considered slow brain waves. Relaxed awareness and daydreaming produce alpha waves.

You are fine if your brainwaves correspond to the behavior or action at hand. Thus, delta waves should be high in amplitude when you are in deep sleep, theta waves high when you let your mind drift, and beta waves dominant when you are paying attention to a task or teacher. However, if the brain produces excessive theta waves when you are trying to concentrate, you have a problem. This is the precise difficulty that children with some forms of ADHD experience. Their brains are producing wave forms associated with daydreaming or drifting off to light sleep when they are trying to concentrate. One way of correcting this mismatch of brain activity to the action required is to give the children drugs, such as Ritalin, that stimulate the central nervous system and help the children focus. A better way to improve the problem is by teaching the children to self-regulate brainwave activity.

Children can learn to regulate their brainwaves by playing a type of video game, but only with their brain. For example, when the brain is producing a healthy pattern, such as reducing the amount of theta-wave activity, balloons move on the computer monitor or a clownlike figure stays out of the water. A brain-controlled Pac-Man game is often a popular and effective reward. Older children and adults are given a simple tone signal when the brain is producing the right waves. Using rewards of sounds and gamelike computer images that provide information about successful brain regulation allows the person to learn what concentration feels like and, better yet, how to sustain that mental state.

The field of brainwave-modification therapy, also called neurotherapy, has experienced impressive growth since the mid-1990s. Therapists can now create full EEG brain maps as a simple in-office procedure to help diagnose and design a treatment program for many troubling conditions. Therapists know, for example, that genetically predisposed alcoholics (and those suffering from other addictions) are often deficient in theta and alpha waves in the back of the brain, the occipital region. For mild blows to the head, the therapist looks for the location of the trauma to the brain. The part of the brain affected by the head injury may not be the point of impact. Most head injuries cause some trauma to the frontal brain regions, and thus, although the impact may have been to the back of the brain, the frontal trauma may be the cause of body pain, mood disorder, and deficiencies of concentration, memory, fine motor skills, sleep, and clarity of speech. Postaccident fibromyalgia (a disorder causing pain and fatigue), for example, is often associated with too much slow activity over the frontal part of the brain, behind the forehead. The predisposition to depression is associated with too much activity over the right front of the brain that is generally not the result of a brain injury but rather is genetic. Many persons suffering from post-traumatic stress disorder (PTSD), a psychological condition resulting from exposure to severe, perhaps life-threatening events, have dysfunctions in the back of the brain and usually a marked reduction in the strength of a specific brainwave.

As can be seen from the above list, some of these problems are genetic, others reflect brain injury, and others may be associated with psychological damage. For the application of brainwave-modification therapies, the origin of the problem is not important. If the condition manifests as an anomalous pattern of brain signals, then that condition is amenable to neurotherapy. Moreover, the outcome of this therapy is usually positive. Plus, once the brainwave problem is fixed, it's fixed. Relapses are rare because the brain functioning has been normalized. This concept of permanence of improvements in brain functioning as a result of neurotherapy can seem odd because of our expectations that continued treatment or at least vigilance is necessary. However, once the brain becomes efficient, those gains are sustained without further treatments unless the person experiences new physical or psychological traumas or disease states. The only exceptions are age-related declines. Later in this book, neurotherapeutic preventative treatment for elderly persons is reviewed. As we get older specific declines in brainwave functioning can be corrected but must be maintained with continuing treatment, usually on a four times per year basis. Neurotherapy thus represents a complete shift in the way we deal with mental problems. No longer do people have to cope with depression for the rest of their lives, relying on mood-altering drugs. Neurotherapy offers hope rather than resignation, feelings of dignity rather than deficiency, empowerment rather than dependence, self-determination as opposed to disappointment.

Here is an illustration of how far the field has developed. When I first saw, or rather smelled, Stacy (no real names of clients are used in this

book) in my waiting room, the verse of a song I used to sing to my kids
came to mind—"and the buzzards in the sky get so drunk they can't fly
from the smell of that good ole mount'n dew." As a general rule, therapists do not see clients when they are intoxicated. However, Stacy's
mother had called and pleaded with us to help her daughter, who was
close to death because of her alcoholism. Stacy tearfully explained that
she desperately needed help, but this morning she simply had to have "a
little something" to help her get to my office. Committed clients have an
excellent chance for full recovery with neurotherapy in combination
with community support programs like Alcoholics Anonymous (AA).
I sensed that Stacy was committed but that she felt powerless. Her alcoholism had been severe for many years, and she had serious medical
problems. Over the previous few weeks her drinking had escalated to
the point where she was continuously inebriated and had experienced
several dangerously close calls when driving.

Stacy had been through many detox/rehab programs, and her physician had tried various regimens of drugs, all to no avail. At the time
when Stacy arrived on my doorstep, neurotherapists had three effective
programs to treat addiction that had been scientifically scrutinized. One
was developed by Peniston. The results of his brainwave treatment,
mentioned before, were published in 1989. Len Ochs had developed a
brain-driving procedure for treating addictions that I learned from him
in that same year.[10] The third treatment method, reported in 1984 by
Margaret Patterson, was a brain-stimulation procedure that has subsequently been developed as an FDA-registered medical device that addicts
can safely self-administer to break the cravings.[11] The details of these neurotherapeutic procedures will be described later; here, I want to highlight
the fact that the procedures had been shown to be safe and effective for
treating addictions such as Stacy's.

I made the ground rules for treatment clear to Stacy: no driving, no
drinking, no hanging out with anyone who was drinking, daily self-
administered treatments with the brain-stimulation device, twice-weekly
neurotherapy treatments in my clinic, daily AA meetings, and permission for me to speak to her mother directly about her treatment
progress. During her next visit, I assured myself that Stacy, now sober,
was serious and that she fully comprehended that her condition was fatal
if she did not stop drinking. Stacy's brain assessment revealed a severe

deficiency of a calming brainwave condition in the back of her brain (elevated beta and reduced theta amplitude). Treatment focused on correcting this deficiency. After thirty-eight treatments Stacy was back in her hometown. Her mother sent me a Christmas card with a kind note. One line read, "It was a blessing to have her at the Christmas dinner table, sober, happy, and with her life back. God bless you."

**FREQUENTLY ASKED QUESTION**

Q: I saw a neurotherapist who said I had to be sober for one month before he would treat me. I can't stop drinking. Can I be treated anyway? A: You need enough sobriety to have a minimally clear head. I have had success with those who could manage to stay sober only a few days. You need to make a full commitment. Go to at least two AA meetings per day, get an AA sponsor, and arrange to start your neurotherapy after two days of complete abstinence.

Over a thousand professionals are credentialed in neurotherapy. Though they are concentrated in the United States, many professionals in other countries offer these treatments. Several universities, principally in the United States, Canada, and the United Kingdom, offer specific training, and many senior therapists provide the necessary supervised training for neurotherapists. Licensed professionals in various health professions—including medicine, psychology, social work, naturopathic and chiropractic medicine—include neurotherapy in their treatment options. Additional information on certification for qualified professionals can be obtained from the Biofeedback Certification Institute of America at www.bcia.org.

Within medicine and psychology, neurotherapy is rapidly gaining wide acceptance. Many physicians specializing in neurology, psychiatry, and internal medicine have been trained in neurotherapy. The major research base of neurotherapy remains in the area of psychology, where most of the important breakthroughs have occurred, and clinical psychologists trained in other forms of therapy have likewise accepted this powerful technology. Associations of professionals with a primary interest in neurotherapy include the International Society for Neuronal Regulation and the Association for Applied Psychophysiology and

Biofeedback. The American Psychological Association recognizes brain-wave biofeedback as an efficacious treatment. Many important peer-reviewed journals publish research in the area of neurotherapy, ensuring that its practice conforms to the highest standards.

I wrote this book to provide you with information that can help you decide whether neurotherapy might be of benefit to you or someone close to you. The chapters have been organized in a step-by-step fashion to offer a full picture of the field, from the equipment in a neurotherapist's office to the different types of brainwaves and locations measured in the brain to the types of disorders that can be treated. Examples of clients who have been treated are discussed throughout the book to show how neurotherapy works in practice.

Based on solid, clinically confirmed scientific research, neurotherapy is emerging as a primary-care alternative to drugs for a wide range of disorders. The focus is on a cure, not just on coping mechanisms. Neurotherapy tackles the problems where they reside—in the brain.

CHAPTER I

# The Basics of Biofeedback

So let's see how neurotherapy would proceed with several very different clients: Jason, a bright and energetic but disheartened child with ADHD; Jane, a chronically worn-out woman hooked on prescription medications that no longer help with her fibromyalgia; and Vincent, the hot-headed, impulsive, and angry victim of traumatic brain injury. After some discussion of the history of brainwave research and clinical applications I review the reasons neurotherapy works to increase brain plasticity.

## A Child with ADHD

The case of Jason, a child with ADHD, is presented in great detail not only to provide an understanding of the process of brainwave biofeedback but also to explain the initial experience with neurotherapy. I begin by describing the first session with Jason, whose father was present because Jason was only twelve years old. I then cover the measurement details, the establishment of client expectations (both child and parent), the development of rapport, the various levels of clinical assessment that the neurotherapist might engage in during the first encounter, and the treatment.

Most children are frightened when they walk into a doctor's office. The sullen, swaggering, rude twelve-year-old boy with the crotch of his jeans down to his knees was no exception. Jason grumpily entered my office, and, despite his heroic efforts to conceal his unease, his eyes widened as he saw the electrodes and other electrical gadgetry in my office. The first thing I told him was "Nothing I do hurts." Kids are not the only ones who become concerned when they see the electrodes that will be attached to their heads. Adults also approach the treatment equipment with a sense of uncertainty. Their initial thought is usually "He's going to give me electroshock therapy." Neurotherapy, though, has nothing to do with giving electric shocks to the brain. The electrodes are for the purpose of measurement only, and I start every new consultation by assuring the client of that.

So what do the electrodes measure? They measure the electrical activity of the inner brain from electrodes attached to the surface of the head with a nonirritating paste the consistency of toothpaste. The electrodes are placed at a series of defined locations for measuring signals across the entire brain. These brain signals are naturally occurring and are in no way stimulated or caused by the electrodes. The signals picked up by the electrodes are displayed on a video monitor. The client feels nothing but can see the electrical activity emitted by the brain on the computer monitors.

I explained to Jason that we would begin by looking at how his brain was functioning. I described how I would use paste the consistency of toothpaste to fasten an electrode attached to a wire to each of his ears and I would also place one on top of his head. I would be moving the electrode on the top of his head to different locations to gain different measurements. Doubt entered Jason's eyes when I told him that, and I reassured him by saying, "You won't feel anything. We are simply measuring the electrical activity of your brain. You'll be able to see your brain activity on the computer monitor." I explained to Jason that the measurements would take ten or fifteen minutes. I promised he would feel nothing, and he could watch the electrical activity coming from his brain on the monitor in front of him. When we were finished, I would remove all the paste from his head and ears and then do some calculations on his measurements. We would then review the information from the brain about his strong areas and areas where he might have some difficulties.

While talking to Jason, I was watching his father out of the corner of my eye. Parents of teenage boys are usually focused on telling me their tales of woe regarding the incorrigibility of their child, their long-suffering tolerance of this behavior, and their willingness to make "one final attempt to help—provided the child will make a serious effort, this time." Parents usually have reasons to be worn out by the behavior of the ADHD child. Jason, for example, had a history of being rude and easily angered. He annoyed his teachers, refused to do his homework, and was unmotivated and highly disruptive in class. He was defiant and oppositional with his family and verbally abusive to his siblings, and he frequently embarrassed his parents in public with his tantrum-like behavior. He was untidy and resisted keeping his room in order. His father abandoned his attempts to get Jason to help around the house as simply too emotionally draining. Needless to say, his school grades were not good, and he was frequently disciplined.

One element of neurotherapy that unsettles parents and older people in general is the notion of changing the way the brain functions. It is completely at odds with what we learned growing up—namely, that the brain you were born with is the brain you must live with. Fortunately, children do not have such hang-ups. They feel comfortable with computers and mind-training concepts. Yet that was not the reason I was talking directly to Jason. His father was trying to enter the conversation to inform me about Jason's problems. Instead I told Jason, "The brain is probably going to tell me everything I need to know about why you are here. If after we go over the results of the brain measurements, there is something I've missed, you can let me know, OK?" I then said to the father, "If there is anything Jason or I miss, please let us know."

Generally, when working with children I engage them in continuous discussion both to relieve their distress and to sustain their attention. I explained to Jason that if he had been brought in with a serious head injury, such as the kind that might occur in a professional hockey game, we would want to measure the signals from all over the brain. To do so we would use a full cap covering the entire head. In his case, however, we would be using the simpler procedure with a single electrode that I had described to him. He would feel nothing, I assured him, because I would only be measuring brain activity, just as his doctor listened to heart activity with a stethoscope. I asked Jason to sit in a chair facing the computer monitor, and then I cleaned his ear lobes with an alcohol wipe with a bit of abrasive to remove oils and surface skin cells. With children

Jason's age, I usually just say that they will feel the cold of the alcohol and the scratching sensation when I clean the scalp. With younger children who still seem frightened I usually say "ouch" when I first touch the ear lobe with the alcohol wipe. Inevitably they laugh and say it did not hurt. I then attached the electrode and wires as I had explained the procedure to Jason.

I asked Jason to open and close his eyes at various times because I needed to determine whether the normal increase in alpha brainwave amplitude with eyes closed dropped rapidly when the eyes were again opened. As discussed in Chapter 2, the alpha response is related to several conditions including traumatic stress and poor visualization skills. The speed of change in alpha amplitude is one of several measures that are important for assessing brain efficiency. I then asked Jason to read for a minute or so to see whether ADHD-like brainwave patterns emerged (some ADHD patterns are observable only when the brain is challenged as when the client is reading or counting backward). I also played a sound that sounds like "shush" to determine exactly how Jason's brain responded to this form of stimulation. If the brain showed positive change when Jason heard the sounds, then I could be confident that his use of this stimulation at home would be beneficial. For example, some sounds have been found to reduce a brainwave amplitude that is associated with focus and attention problems. (These sounds and other adjunctive treatments meant for home use are described later in this chapter.)

Using the procedures that I have developed, the measurement phase is short. The measurements require two and a half minutes of recording on top of the head, one minute at the back, forty-five seconds over each of the two frontal lobes, and eighty seconds of recording over the middle of the front part of the brain. This adds up to only six minutes and twenty seconds of data gathering, but with moving electrodes, printing the data, and chatting with the child, the procedure usually takes fifteen minutes or so in total.

While the measurements were in progress, I spoke softly to Jason, placing my hand on his shoulder and reinforcing his cooperative participation. I was also instructing his father, to some extent, in that he observed me directing Jason in a firm but kind manner. In general, I engage the child but do not permit disruptive behavior. Occasionally, therapists run into parenting situations that are out of control. Some are minor, such as a parent constantly interrupting with admonishments to the child to "sit up" or "pay attention." Others reflect serious family problems, such as when a parent stops the session because the child doesn't want to continue. I am reminded of a six-year-old child who couldn't read because his mother said he did not have to learn if he did not want to and, more serious, a child who was threatened with being put up for adoption if she did not behave properly. Such situations obviously require family therapy in addition to neurotherapy. Fortunately, in Jason's situation, the father, although angry and worn out, understood the need for parental authority and responsibility.

After taking all the measurements, I printed out the data and made some calculations to determine the areas of Jason's brain that showed problematical activity. I go over my calculations with clients in detail to verify that the information I have gained about their condition matches their experiences and is the reason they are seeking or have been brought to me for treatment. This part concerns mostly the parents, but the child is kept as strongly engaged as possible during the review. I explain that some brainwaves are associated with slow activity in the brain, such as daydreaming; other brainwaves are associated with brain efficiency; others with trauma; and still others with processing information. (The details of brainwave assessment are covered in Chapter 2.)

Because children with ADHD often hear bad news when they go to physicians and psychologists, school counselors and teachers, I always start with the positive features found in the brain map, and good signs can always be found. In Jason's case, I was lucky to see that his brain showed what I call the "artist's signature." The artist's signature is a brainwave pattern that is correlated with a proclivity for artistic, spatial, and musical creativity. "Jason, look at this. Do you like to draw or build things or write or play music? This is the artist's signature in the brain." I could tell by the look on his father's face and by Jason's smile that I had guessed right. "He's always drawing and building stuff," said Dad enthusiastically. "He used to be crazy about Legos and now he builds models—he also takes apart a lot of things and forgets to put them back together." He looked at me curiously. "How did you know that about Jason?"

I responded, "The brain tells us everything," a concept I repeat over and over during the first session with a client. As I review in detail in

Chapter 2, the patterning of brainwaves is directly associated with symptoms. By interpreting these patterns, the neurotherapist is able to describe the client's symptoms in detail without any information from the client. I showed Jason and Dad the artist's signature in the brain activity. It appears as a large increase in the alpha brainwave when the client closes his eyes. "Jason," I said, "that is an extremely valuable skill to have. Good artists, architects, choreographers, and fiction writers have that signature, and so do fine cabinetmakers and good mechanics."

After reviewing the areas of brain functioning that are within normal limits, I home in on the reason the child has been brought to my office. Jason had a severe case of a form of ADHD that I find more often in males than in females. In Jason's case, the indicator of the disorder was an excessive amount of slow-frequency theta waves over the top of his brain. The excessive amplitude became even more pronounced when he read. This form of ADHD was identified by Christopher Mann and his colleagues at the University of Tennessee in a 1992 study of twenty-five male children.[1] This frustrating form of ADHD seems to worsen the more the child attempts to focus. It often goes undetected if the brainwave data are obtained only under resting conditions. At rest the brainwaves do not show any unusual patterning, but when the child reads or counts backward, the brain produces brainwaves associated with the early stages of sleep.

As I showed this pattern to Jason and his father, I asked the boy, "In class, do you have problems staying with the teacher?" Jason nodded. "Do you find yourself thinking about other things when the teacher is talking?" He kept on nodding. "When you read, do you sometimes find that when you get to the end of the paragraph or page you have forgotten what you just read?" His face was starting to crack. "When taking a test, do you sometimes forget the question when you want to start the answer?" He was getting upset, but I had one more question. "Do you find that sometimes you feel that you have to move, tap your feet or hands?" Jason was making a strong effort not to cry, so I addressed my remarks to the father. "With conditions like this, kids just give up. They are told that they are not trying, yet despite their best efforts they still can't do it. The vicious thing about this disorder is that the harder he tries, the worse it gets."

I explained that this condition could be corrected. The same electrodes used in the assessment would be placed on Jason during treatment sessions. The electrodes were again for measurement only, and Jason would not feel anything. I explained that basically Jason would be "playing a video game with only your brain. You don't touch anything. You simply try to get into the mental state that will cause pictures on the computer monitor to move. As you play you will discover how to control your thoughts to be successful at the game." We set up the treatment so that when Jason made his slow brainwaves decline, an animated video character (Pac-Man) moved on the screen. Through concentrating, Jason gradually learned to reduce the amplitude of his slow theta waves to the normal range. Children are usually interested in playing the many video games associated with biofeedback. They become skilled at moving the game icons. As the game proceeds, a score tallies, for example, the number of dots Pac-Man eats up.

An important concept in this training is that the game gets more difficult as the child becomes more skilled. As Jason got better at getting high scores in the game, I made the game more difficult. To explain the reason for this procedure, I usually use the example of a high jumper. When the athlete first starts training, he sets the bar at a level he can clear most of the time. As he gets better, he challenges himself by raising the bar. By continuing to raise the bar he learns how to jump over higher levels. Jason understood this concept. As he got better at controlling his brain, I made it harder for him to move Pac-Man because it required a larger change in his brainwaves. This is the concept of *threshold,* which is the level of brain activity required to receive feedback. In Jason's case, the threshold was constantly changed during each session so that Pac-Man moved about 70 percent of the time.

Most neurotherapists try to make use of every moment of contact with children during treatment. While moving the electrodes, I chat about sports they play, favorite pastimes, and things they collect. I have many objects in my office, including old bottles, arrowheads, semiprecious stones, fossils, sharks' teeth, and old money. The children usually become intrigued by these items, and I then introduce "Dr. Swingle's Treasure Chest," which contains similar items but no toys or candy. I tell the children that at the end of every session they can take one of the items from the treasure chest. These items not only are a reward but also support the educational model of the treatment, a process that is critical when working with children. After brain treatment children are intellectually sharp. The session they have just completed was directed at increasing focus and concentration so the slow brainwave frequencies are lowered and the fast frequencies are strengthened. These brainwave changes increase the children's understanding and retention of the information relevant to the treasure-chest items. The items in the treasure chest are all labeled with a short, informative description. Also on the wall above the chest are world maps, geological calendars, and sample charts so the children can identify, date, and locate any item in the chest. Because of their heightened mental state they do not forget this information. Often they bring these items to school for show-and-tell, frequently startling teachers with the breadth of their knowledge about the items. Most children Jason's age are too threatened ("too old") to admit to wanting to dig about in the chest for a treasure, but chatting with me about these interesting items motivates them to participate in this important component of treatment.

Neurotherapists usually prescribe some home treatments for clients to help with the brainwave changes. In Jason's case, I prescribed a light stimulation device that would suppress the slow amplitude while he was reading or doing other mental activities. The lights are usually light emitting diodes (LEDs) that are attached to eyeglass frames. In general, the form of light stimulation that is useful in neurotherapy is a repetitive flash that triggers the brain to produce an EEG response at the same frequency.[2] For Jason, using the light stimulation while he read would likely help him because the pulsating lights would stimulate brainwave activity consistent with concentration.

**FREQUENTLY ASKED QUESTION**

Q: I have seen advertisements for devices that flash lights in your eyes to help you relax. Do these things really work?

A: Visual (and auditory) stimulation at the correct frequencies can increase the strength of brainwaves that can help you relax or concentrate. We use many such devices in the treatment of a variety of disorders.

I also prescribed a recorded audio CD developed in our clinic that Jason could use while doing homework. The sound on the CD was a filtered "pink noise" that sounds like running water, but it contained subliminal sounds at various frequencies that suppressed the slow-frequency brainwave amplitude and thereby helped Jason concentrate and retain information. I had tested the sound on the CD during Jason's assessment. The sound had immediately suppressed the problematic slow frequency by 15.6 percent, so I knew it would work.

Jason needed twenty-six sessions over eight months to learn to normalize the slow brain activity. He soon reported that, with the exception of one C, his grades were "great." His relationship with his father was much improved. However, Jason was still a teenager—a condition that cannot be treated with neurotherapy.[3]

## A Holistic Intervention Plan

A theme that I stress throughout this book is that brainwave biofeedback is not a stand-alone treatment. One can markedly improve the poor functioning of the brain of an ADHD child, for example, but still not see important changes in the child's performance, family relationships, or personal sense of worth. Children with ADHD often develop major psychosocial dysfunctions because of their struggles with the disorder. To help the child with ADHD, the neurotherapist pays attention to family dynamics; the parenting skills of the parents; the self-esteem of the child; the child's relationship with peers, siblings, and teachers; and the child's interests, skills, and concerns. In other words, the neurotherapist deals with the problem holistically, and the emphasis is on self-regulation. Every effort is made to avoid pathologizing the child's problems.

Disorders like ADHD are thus not just problems for the individual but should be considered family disorders. Most problems—including alcoholism, depression, anxiety, chronic pain, traumatic brain injury, and age-related declines in memory—generally affect an individual's entire family and friends. Further, tending to the neurological problem may not resolve the associated psychological issues, which can continue to have debilitating effects on the sufferer. Therefore, clients and their families generally can benefit from complementary therapies to deal with the social and psychological "baggage" associated with such disorders.

ADHD and other consequences of brain inefficiencies can seriously disrupt the way a family functions, as was the case with Jason's family.

Resentment, anger, defiance, and disappointment are all direct consequences of the ADHD child's inability to maintain focus. Being told that
they are not working or are not trying or are lazy, when in fact they are
doing their best, inevitably leads the children to conclude that they are
stupid, worthless, and unlikable. Frequent giving up, defiance, and
other forms of acting out are vain efforts to protect themselves from
their core emotional belief about themselves. And self-loathing is not
too strong a term to describe the emotional pain of these children.

Because of the emotional consequences of the ADHD symptoms,
family dynamics are critical. The frustration, anger, hostility, emotional
volatility, defiance, and other negative dynamics usually must be addressed
in addition to improving brain functioning. Most prominent clinicians and
researchers in the area of the treatment of ADD and ADHD stress that for
neurotherapy to have long-lasting results the family problems also must be
addressed. These dynamics are complex. A disruptive family environment
can cause attention problems in any school-age child, and inappropriate
parental behavior can worsen the child's ADHD problems. Parents get
angry with the hyperactive child, feel that the child is defiant, and experience feelings of failure as a parent. Parents' beliefs that their child is "not
trying" or is "lazy" can cause that very behavior because the child may simply give up. Neurotherapists always advise parents to attend to parenting
skills. They often recommend family therapy or some of the excellent
books on raising children with ADHD, such as Vincent Monastra's helpful
*Parenting the Child with ADHD: 10 Lessons That Medicine Cannot Teach*.[4]

Jason's parents benefited from a few sessions of family therapy, which
helped them to improve their effectiveness as parents of a child whose
school experiences had been humiliating and harmful to his self-concept.
The problem can be much more complicated with adults. Just imagine if
Jason were forty years old before he came for treatment. He might well be
alcoholic or addicted to some other substance, engaged in other harmful
behaviors, at a career dead-end, unsuccessful at relationships, angry,
depressed, and convinced that he was a defective human being. Once his
neurological functioning improved, the older Jason might still require
some psychological assistance to overcome the years of learning to hide
from his feelings of inadequacy.

Joel and Judith Lubar report that adults with ADD are likely to have
reactive depression because of repeated failures and inability to meet
their own, often unrealistic, standards. Indeed, between 70 and 90

percent of children with ADHD continue to experience significant problems in adulthood.[5] Neurotherapists have known for some time that a far greater percentage of children with ADHD than those without that condition develop problems with alcoholism and drug addiction. These patterns were reported in 2001 by Maria Sullivan of the Columbia Presbyterian Medical Center in New York.[6] Sullivan points out that about 50 percent of adults with ADHD symptoms have a substance-use disorder, including more than 50 percent greater nicotine dependence compared with the general population. Individuals with continuing ADHD symptoms, she reports, abuse drugs earlier, use them longer, and are more likely to progress from alcohol abuse to other medical and nonmedical drug abuse than individuals without ADHD symptoms.

---

**FREQUENTLY ASKED QUESTION**

Q: My brother is a drug addict and tells me that his addiction was caused by his ADHD. Is this true?

A: Many adults with untreated ADHD develop problems with drugs. Often this occurs because the ADHD leads to failures that in turn lead to attempts to escape the negative feelings about being a failure through the use of alcohol or drugs.

---

Another aspect of this issue is also important. Consider an older Jason, in a troubled marriage, who is in marital counseling with his wife. The counseling does not seem to be going anywhere, and Jason and his wife are likely to end up among the greater than 50 percent of couples who fail in marital counseling. Why? In this case the marital counselor may be missing an essential part of the problem. Family disorder can stem from adult ADHD, which manifests itself in alcohol abuse, anger problems, and career failure. The efficacy of marital counseling is likely to increase if all the facets of the problem are treated—that is, if the brain inefficiencies are corrected with neurotherapy and the interpersonal problems are resolved in marital counseling. Jason might also benefit from some individual therapy focused on important life changes, including career counseling and treatment for self-destructive addictive behavior.

Our clinic works closely with a number of family and couple counselors who find that neurotherapy can be beneficial for a different reason.

An area in the brain called the anterior cingulate cortex is associated with uncompromising behavior. When "hot," this area can be associated with obsessive, compulsive, stubborn, and self-absorbed behavior. This area is often found to be overactive in defiant children and children with autism. When this area is hot in one or both parties to a marriage, insufficient cooperative and compromising behavior can lead to significant discord. Family counselors often refer such "stuck" couples for assessment. If this area of the brain is functioning inefficiently, a neurotherapist can normalize it in the affected spouse and then send the couple back to continue with the marital counseling.

## A Woman with Chronic Problems

As a general rule, the more chronic the disorder, the more supporting therapies will be needed. In this context, the term *chronic* refers to the length of time the client has endured a disorder, not the severity of the disorder. Chronicity is important because over time the sufferer develops dysfunctional habits to deal with the disorder and its social and psychological consequences. The young Jason's ADHD would not be considered chronic, whereas the older Jason's condition would be chronic and therefore require additional therapeutic help. Chronicity leads to despair, as the case of Jane suggests.

Jane was a slight woman in her late fifties who seemed meek, in pain, and chronically depressed. She appeared as though she felt cold, and tears started down her cheeks as soon as she sat down. She looked around my office at my odd assortment of "artifacts" and smiled. I said, "It's an incurable disease—I collect everything." That lightened the strain on her face a little. Jane proceeded to tell me that a friend of hers had been to see me and had derived remarkable benefits from neurotherapy. I asked Jane whether she knew what I did, and she said that she knew little but thought that I stimulated the brain. Like Jason, Jane initially thought I would pass an electrical current through her brain in an office version of electroshock therapy. This mistaken belief often has one of two causes (or both causes). First, when clients see the electrodes, they immediately think that they are meant to deliver electricity rather than to measure physiological activity. Second, adult clients referred by other clients often receive a confused description of the treatment. Neuro-feedback does not involve any electrical stimulation. However, for some conditions such as depression, addiction, anxiety, pain, and sleep problems, I often prescribe cranial microamperage stimulation (known by the acronym CES) for home use, as described in Chapter 4.

Clients like Jane are both good news and bad news for neurotherapists. The good news is that, having been referred by a satisfied client, Jane was less skeptical about treatment and more inclined to follow the therapy recommendations than someone who had no connection to neurotherapy. The bad news is that, being middle-aged, she probably had a chronic condition and therefore had likely become accustomed to her pain, had become addicted or habituated to medications, and felt pessimistic and scared about her future. She had probably tried many treatments, adjusted her lifestyle to accommodate her limitations, and become emotionally dependent on a health provider, typically a physician, but often a psychologist or counselor. Regrettably, such health care providers are usually committed to their approach. They may resist any treatment options that are unfamiliar, thinking the practitioner is holding out false hope to the patient.

Jane wanted sympathy, so my first job was to let her describe her problems. She had a long history of depression, feelings of inadequacy, lack of energy and motivation, and conditions associated with general anxiety. She went on to explain that although heavily medicated she did not find relief and presently she felt hopeless and defeated. After sympathetically listening to her for a while, I engaged her in committing to a course of treatment that was focused on improvement of her condition, not just on coping. This is an important issue. To resolve chronic conditions, a client has to accept that mood-altering and pain-relief medications will eventually be eliminated or, at least, markedly reduced. Rehabilitation facilities have many clients who are treated for addiction to prescription medications. Radio talk-show host Rush Limbaugh's addiction to pain medications is well known. Treatment of clients like Jane entails significant psychological counseling as well as neurotherapy in order to help them eliminate their reliance on drugs.

Jane's brain assessment revealed a pattern typically associated with fibromyalgia. This connective-tissue disorder causes the client to feel pain in many parts of the body. The pain often moves around. Sleep is usually seriously disrupted, and chronic fatigue is common. Many more women than men are affected by this disorder. Fibromyalgia appears to be related to physical trauma, such as that resulting from an automobile accident, viral infection (such as a serious flu), or severe psychological stress.

Jane had excessive slow-frequency theta brainwave amplitude in the front part of the brain. The brainwave signature for this condition was reported in 1998 by Stuart Donaldson, clinic director at Myosymmetries in Calgary, Alberta, and his colleagues.[7] In addition, Barbara Westmoreland of the Mayo Clinic reported in 1993 that increased frontal slow-frequency brainwave amplitude is found with other viral infections such as measles.[8] Typically, these clients show excessive theta and alpha amplitudes and deficient beta amplitude. These disturbances in brainwave activity are consistent with patients' reports of fatigue, pain, sleep disturbance, and cognitive fogginess. In addition to the brainwave slowing, Jane also had deficient slow brainwave amplitude in the back of the brain and a frontal-lobe disparity that indicated depression. I told Jane that she experienced "fibrofog," sleep disturbance, and depression and showed her the areas of brain activity that needed help.

**FREQUENTLY ASKED QUESTION**

Q: My wife says that her doctor told her that fibromyalgia is caused by stress and that there is no cure. This seems contradictory to me. Can fibromyalgia be treated?

A: Stress doesn't actually cause anything. It can only increase the likelihood of occurrence. Treatment of fibromyalgia is possible through neurotherapeutic correction of the neurological predisposition plus treatment for stress management.

I introduce Jane's case at this point to correct any notions that neurotherapy is a magic bullet. Jason's condition was a simple case of ADHD that responded quickly to neurotherapy. The psychological component of his treatment focused largely on encouraging Jason's father to have realistic expectations and to reestablish Jason's belief in himself. Once the functioning of the problematical areas in Jason's brain were normalized, the developmental process kicked in, and Jason became increasingly capable of capitalizing on his considerable intellectual strengths.

Jane, however, was a much more complicated client than Jason, even though the total number of neurotherapy sessions required to normalize brain activity was about the same. Jane needed the courage to break her dependencies on medications; on sympathetic but enabling health care providers; on pity as a unifying factor in her relationships; and on seeing herself as a deficient person. Also, her pace of treatment was slower than Jason's. Once Jane's sleeping improved and her pain was somewhat reduced, sessions were spread out to once per month to allow her time to gradually reduce her medications and to introduce new activities into her life.

Jane was not sure when she became aware of her fibromyalgia condition. She did not recall any physical injury, but she did recall a rather serious "cold." She admitted that she had been sexually assaulted by a family member when she was a young child. Jane's situation is not uncommon with women who develop fibromyalgia. They often report severe psychological trauma and an episode of a viral infection. Jane benefited from a few psychotherapy sessions. Her major psychological "breakthrough" came when she saw herself as a rape victim rather than as a shame-ridden person who felt responsible for the sexual abuse.

Jane finished treatment several years ago, and I still hear from her from time to time. She is doing remarkably well, has become employed, and refers many clients to me. She has finally stopped taking all mood-altering and pain medications and recently got married.

### The Origins of Neurotherapy

Thousands of years ago, the healers of the day made tiny holes in the skulls of people with problems, apparently in an effort to allow troubling spirits to be released from the head. This surgical procedure, called trepanation, was quite in vogue. At various archeological digs on different continents, 30 to 40 percent of the recovered skulls show evidence of trepanation. Jim Robbins, in his book *A Symphony in the Brain,* reports that at one site near Cuzco, Peru, 40 percent of three thousand mummies had trepanned skulls and apparently 65 percent of these "surgery" patients survived the operation.[9]

Neurotherapy began with the discovery that the brain both produced electrical signals and responded to electrical stimulation. Beginning around

1875, scientists including Richard Caton, Charles Beevor, Korbinian Brodmann, Paul Broca, Carl Wernicke, Victor Horsley, Gustav Fritsch, Leon Chaffee, Rudolf Hess, and Eduard Hertzig mapped areas of the animal and human brain that were associated with various movements, behaviors, feelings, sensations, and thoughts. Their work was based on previous discoveries that specific areas of the brain were associated with specific functions.

The seminal work on the mapping of the human brain was done by Canadian neurosurgeon Wilder Penfield, who in 1928 became the director of the Neurological Institute at McGill University in Montreal. During brain surgery with conscious patients, Penfield electrically stimulated areas of the brain. He found areas that were associated with body movement, sensation and perception, and memories. His patients heard sounds and voices, felt various body sensations, smelled odors, and gave involuntary utterances all in response to stimulating electrical current applied to various locations in the brain. Penfield mapped the motor cortex, the area of the brain associated with the movement of specific body parts.[10] This map is called a homunculus, or "little man," because the specific brain areas associated with specific body parts are ordered systematically from feet to head on the cortex. The homunculus is used today to guide both neurosurgery and the placement of electrodes for neurofeedback with brain-injured clients whose ability to move their body has been affected by their injury.

An area of research related to brain mapping, but with a more ominous potential, is the direct stimulation of the brain to elicit specific effects. In a 1956 issue of *Scientific American,* psychologist James Olds reported his discovery of a pleasure zone in the brain.[11] He found that animals with electrodes implanted in this zone would self-administer electrical pulses to this area several thousand times per hour, ignoring food when hungry, even highly-favored food. This procedure was extended to humans when Carl Sem-Jacobsen and Arne Torkildsen, two Norwegian researchers at the Gauster Mental Hospital in Oslo, implanted electrodes in the pleasure centers of the brains of mental patients. Some patients controlled the electrodes so as to stimulate the pleasure centers to the extent of bringing on convulsions.[12]

A number of researchers later found that electrical stimulation of the area of the brain called the amygdala can elicit rage or fear, plus aggressive or timid behavior in animals such as cats and monkeys. The amygdala is important in emotional regulation. Apparently, the amygdala also processes socially relevant emotional information. José Delgado, who at the time was director of the Neuropsychiatry Department at Yale University School of Medicine, dramatically demonstrated the potential of brain-stimulation technology when he implanted a radio-controlled brain-stimulation device in a bull's brain. According to a sensational article in the *New York Times,* Delgado entered a bullring in Spain with his red cape and portable radio transmitter, facing a charging bull. When Delgado activated the stimulator the bull stopped charging and timidly withdrew.[13]

In addition to brain mapping and the direct stimulation of the brain, a third avenue of research related to neurotherapy is the exterior measurement of the brain's electrical activity. In 1875, Richard Caton found that electrical activity could be recorded from the surface of the exposed brains of animals. Activities of various sorts produced different forms of electrical activity. In the 1920s, Hans Berger, a German psychiatrist, expanded on Caton's work when he discovered that the electrical activity of the brain could be measured with skin-surface electrodes placed on the scalp rather than on the exposed brain. He obtained many electrical recordings, which he called electroencephalograms (EEGs), from his son, his daughter, and later his psychiatric patients. He found that a slow-frequency wave, now called "alpha," in the range of about 10 cycles per second (10 Hertz, Hz) was predominant when the client was at rest, whereas faster frequencies were observed when the brain was challenged (for example, when he asked his daughter to do a mathematical calculation).

### SOME POSSIBLE BRAINWAVE EFFECTS

| TOO MUCH | BRAINWAVE | TOO LITTLE |
|---|---|---|
| Mental fog, pain | Delta | Poor sleep |
| Can't stay focused | Theta | Can't relax |
| Can't finish projects, can't sleep | Alpha | Mental chatter |
| Anxiety | Beta | Can't concentrate |

In the 1960s psychologists Neil Miller and Leo DiCara, who were at Yale and Rockefeller universities, published several papers showing that animals and humans could control activities of the autonomic nervous system such as heart rate and blood pressure.[14] These finding were quite revolutionary given the physiological theories at the time. Physiological systems such as blood pressure, heart rate, and body temperature were assumed to be homeostatic in nature: when you become anxious, your heart rate accelerates, and your blood pressure rises. But if one could directly influence the physiological systems associated with anxiety, then one might be able to reduce feelings of anxiety, for example, by reducing the physiological correlates of those states. Researchers following the seminal work of DiCara and Miller did exactly that and found that profound states of body quiet could be achieved with autonomic biofeedback; the systems that could be affected included muscle tension, heart rate, surface body temperature, and the electrical conductivity of the skin. I discuss these forms of biofeedback in detail later in this book. The first brainwave biofeedback was reported in 1934 by two researchers at Cambridge University in England who were replicating Berger's findings. These researchers found that they could increase their alpha brainwave rhythm at will. Alpha can be increased in amplitude quite readily by imagining as vividly as one can a sailing ship disappearing over the horizon.

Thirty years after Berger reported his findings, scientists began to explore the clinical uses of biofeedback of the brain. At the University of Chicago, psychologist Joe Kamiya, following the lead of Berger and the Cambridge University scientists, explored the effects of EEG changes on consciousness. Kamiya, whose work with alpha waves had begun in the mid-1950s, discovered that profound states of mental quiet could be achieved with alpha-frequency brainwave biofeedback.[15] (His work is often remembered as the development of "technological Zen.") At Sepulveda Veterans Administration Hospital in California, Barry Sterman found that cats could learn to increase (or decrease) brainwave activity if given a food reward. He also discovered that cats that had been trained to increase the amplitude of particular brainwaves (the sensory motor rhythm—SMR) were resistant to seizures when exposed to a seizure-inducing compound found in rocket fuels. (I examine Sterman's work in detail in Chapter 2.)

Since the late 1960s, research in psychoneurophysiology has been increasing. Unfortunately, much of what people know about the field is the narrow segment of biofeedback used for mental and physical quieting.

It was thought that quieting the mind and the body would have profound beneficial effects on mind/body healing through the reduction of the adverse effects of stress in general. Although true, this restricted view wrongly led many people to the conclusion that all types of biofeedback were simply exotic and expensive forms of relaxation and technology-assisted meditation. Although often facilitating and accelerating the calming process, in general biofeedback did not necessarily accomplish any more profound healing than relaxing the mind/body with meditation, muscle relaxation, hypnosis, and the like.

In contrast, neurotherapy has emerged as a powerful primary-care alternative in a wide range of areas. Using a variety of specific techniques in addition to biofeedback, neurotherapists developed effective, safe, and cost-efficient treatments for many psychophysiological conditions ranging from seizure disorders and head injuries to psychological conditions, including profound depression, obsessive-compulsive disorders, learning problems, and severe post-traumatic stress disorders. Clinical research supporting neurotherapy can be found in many scientific journals, including the specialized *Journal of Neurotherapy* and *Applied Psychophysiology and Biofeedback,* both available on the Internet. The three conditions for which there is the most research establishing the efficacy of neurofeedback, including controlled studies published in peer-reviewed journals, are epilepsy, depression, and ADHD. For many other conditions, there are clinical reports of successful interventions, and this applied work is moving ahead.

## The Plasticity of the Brain: Expanding Boundaries

Another exciting avenue of research, enriching the brain's general capabilities, has tremendous potential. Traditionally, people have been taught that they have to live with the limitations they were born with. If you are born with an IQ of 85, then you have that level of intelligence for life. Another old belief is that brain damage is permanent because the brain cannot regenerate. Yet researchers have established that these ideas are wrong. The mind is capable of astounding regeneration, growth, and change. Most of the brain's systems are plastic, meaning that they can be modified by learning, including the training that takes place with neurotherapy. In addition, such experiences change the brain's cellular structure through the branching of neuronal axons and new synaptic growth at the point at which the brain cells communicate.[16] Researchers have shown that the IQ increases by 10 to 12 points with routine brain-wave biofeedback; this research confirms that structural changes take place in the brain as a result of neurotherapy.[17]

Even with conditions that have a strong genetic component, the evidence clearly indicates that learning factors are implicated in their manifestation. Geneticist John Cairns and his colleagues at Harvard University found that some gene mutations were adaptive (that is, not random).[18] Biological researchers have been reporting for decades that genes are not self-determined but require environmental signals for activation. Identical-twin studies show that conditions like depression, schizophrenia, ADHD, and alcoholism have a genetic link. For example, when schizophrenia is found in one twin, the identical twin has a 50 percent likelihood of developing it too—even if they are raised apart. The equally important aspect of this research is that 50 percent of the twins do not show evidence of schizophrenia, a finding that underscores the critical role played by experiential factors in addition to basic genetic predispositions. Our potential for recovery and growth is not biologically predetermined. We are not simply a slave to our genes. The general rule of thumb is that if there is structure, then function can be restored. If all nerve cells have been destroyed, there is no structure and hence no electrical signal to be measured and trained. Usually there is some structure, a few neurons still firing, and therefore a chance for improvement with neurotherapy.

**FREQUENTLY ASKED QUESTION**

Q: I had a stroke four years ago. I made a good recovery during the first year or so but little since. My physiotherapist said that most of the recovery takes place in the first two years and little thereafter. Is there any reason for optimism four years after the stroke?

A: Before the development of neurotherapy, recovery from brain injury usually reached a plateau after eighteen months. Now, however, we have learned how to nudge the brain toward further recovery, so significant gains are often possible long after a stroke.

The brain is nearly always capable of recovery and growth. Mark Rosenzweig's research at the University of California at Berkeley showed that brain-cell populations are affected dramatically by experience.[19] At a fundamental level, Bruce Lipton has shown that genes do not determine behavior but must be "turned on" by experience, thoughts, or emotions.[20] The scientific data suggest that the brain can learn to change its "biological wiring" patterns and function in an improved manner. Brain-injured patients can recover the function of muscles years after the presumed loss of the potential for recovery.

Robert Thatcher, professor at the University of South Florida College of Medicine, summarizes many of the important issues in traumatic brain injury (TBI) in his review article in *Clinical Electroencephalography*. Thatcher points out that TBI virtually always damages the frontal areas in the brain, so people with TBI have serious problems with executive functions such as planning, managing anger, and emotional and impulse control.[21] Many death-row inmates show evidence of frontal-lobe damage. James Evans, professor at the University of South Carolina, created brain maps for twenty death-row inmates.[22] He found that all had evidence of brain abnormalities and most had a concentration of these dysfunctions in the front (behind the forehead) and, in particular, the right frontal areas of the brain. This concentration of brain dysfunction in the frontal regions suggests a brain injury because the frontal lobes are the most vulnerable to damage. The Brain Injury Association of America estimates that 2 percent of the population is disabled from TBI.[23] In addition to mood disorders and anger problems, the common effects of TBI are problems with memory, agitation, anxiety, fatigue, comprehension, perseveration, motivation, reasoning, problem solving, rate of activity, and concentration. The following case shows how neurotherapy can help brains recover from head injuries.

Vincent was yelling at our receptionist when I first encountered him. He was angry about being asked to pay for his first visit before he saw me. (We occasionally ask clients to prepay when there is only one receptionist in the clinic and the visit occurs just before lunchtime or closing time.) Vincent was irate, claiming we were interested only in his money, asking why he should pay before he received services, accusing the receptionist of being incompetent, to mention but a few issues. I glanced at the appointment schedule and saw that he was scheduled for a full, nineteen-location brain map. Going directly to full brain mapping usually means that the referring doctor has identified the problem as a brain injury or stroke. Vincent later told me of a severe head injury he sustained when working as a longshoreman.

Neurotherapists find that brain-injured clients are often easily distracted so, rather than arguing with Vincent, I said, "Relax, Vincent, you're going to blow a gasket."

"Who are you?" he asked in a hostile tone.

"You came here to get your head examined, and I'm the guy who is going to do it."

"You Dr. Swingle?"

"Paul Swingle, glad to meet you, Vincent. Come into my office. You can pay me later. But if you give me a hard time, I'll charge you double!"

Vincent started laughing at this point. "I certainly need my head examined," he said as he followed me into my office.

Even after he sat down, though, he continued to be hostile, complaining about doctors, how he had been treated, how he could not be sure that I wasn't a phony, how he was not going to put up with any disrespect from me or my staff, and so on. When he slowed down, I softly said, "Vincent, you came to me for help. Head injuries always make people a bit crazy. You do and say things you don't want to do or say. People start avoiding you. They are afraid of your potential for violence. They don't like to be around you, so you feel miserable, depressed, and confused. Right?" Vincent nodded. "Give this a chance. Keep an open mind—our success rate with helping people like you is excellent."

"You're right," he said, calming down. "Last week I was walking behind a beautiful woman and grabbed her ass on a crowded street. I was with someone who yelled at me that I couldn't just grab people or bother them. Luckily, he dragged me away, and the woman just stood there yelling at me, so nothing else happened. I don't remember why I did it—it seemed like a good idea. My buddy kept asking me if I knew it was wrong." He shook his head. "It really didn't seem wrong at the time." This is a good example of disinhibition after injury to the frontal lobes, where our social conscience resides.

I explained how neurotherapy works and reviewed the brain-mapping procedure. Full nineteen-site brain maps provide much more data about brain functioning than the five-site assessment used with clients

like Jason and Jane. For brain injury, the full map is essential, in particular to detect how different parts of the brain are communicating with
each other. I asked Vincent to sit in the chair next to the recording
instruments (the EEG). As I picked up the full electrode cap, preparing
to place it over his head, he jumped up and yelled, "You're not putting
that [expletive] thing on my head!"

I asked, "Why not?"

"You're going to give me electric shock. You want to shock my brain.
I like my brain the way it is."

Even though I had reviewed the brain-assessment process in detail,
Vincent still retained the idea that the purpose of the electrodes was to
shock his brain. The electrode cap used for brain mapping does look a
bit daunting. It covers the entire head from just above the eyebrows to
the upper part of the neck. Flaps go over the ears, and more than twenty
wires flow from the cap to a cable that is plugged into a large gray case
with lots of switches, lights, and connectors. Straps go under the chin to
hold the cap securely in place. Even when clients have been assured that
they will not feel any electrical stimulation because there is none to be
felt, the process of placing and securing the cap and preparing the electrode sites frequently upsets them. I reminded Vincent that I had promised no electrical current would be delivered to his head. I then asked
him whether he had ever had an electrocardiograph (ECG or EKG)
taken of his heart. He replied that he had, so I asked him whether he
felt any electrical stimulation during the measurements. He said no. I
assured him that the principle of the EEG was the same as the principle
of the ECG, in that the electrodes simply measure the physiological
activity of the brain. He would feel nothing. Vincent sat down again, and
I proceeded to secure the cap. He did, however, continue to seek reas-
surance that he was not going to be shocked.

While preparing the multiple sites for measuring the brain's electrical
activity, I have to use a blunt tube on the end of a syringe to squirt a pasty
solution (an electrode gel) that conducts electricity into the space between
the scalp and the electrode. This is not an uncomfortable experience, but
two electrode sites on the forehead can be sensitive when rubbed with the
blunt tube at the end of the "needle." After inserting the gel, it is usually
necessary to rub gently with the blunt end of the tube to move hair out of
the way to ensure a good contact between scalp and electrode.

Vincent had fifteen treatment sessions before he stopped worrying about me electrically stimulating his brain. This obsessiveness, or perseveration, is common in TBI, where short-term memory is compromised: patients get an idea in their heads and can't get it out. The effects of brain injury on concentration and memory have been well documented. For example, physicians at University Hospital in Groeningen, the Netherlands, showed that one year after the head injury 84 percent of their patients still reported symptoms, the most common being irritability, forgetfulness, poor concentration, and fatigue.[24]

In the end, Vincent needed nearly fifty neurotherapy treatments, plus a few psychotherapy sessions, to provide balance in his emotional life and improve the efficiency of his cognitive functioning. Since doing the training, he has been employed at the same job for over two years and has reunited with his wife after having been separated. Vincent still must pay attention to his volatile mood states, but he claims that his anger and rage are well under control. I met Vincent a year after he ended treatment, and he told me that he was thankful that he received the neurotherapy. He recognized that, without the training, his anger and rage could have increased, and he could have seriously harmed someone.

One of the major contributions of neurotherapy to the treatment of TBI is to correctly identify injured areas of the brain. Thatcher, mentioned previously for his work on frontal-lobe involvement in TBI, is one of the pioneers in the development of databases for identifying TBI. The data show that conventional visual EEG and visual magnetic resonance imaging (MRI) procedures commonly used in hospitals correctly identify TBI in fewer than 20 percent of the cases.[25] However, Kirtley Thornton and Dennis Carmody of the Center for Health Psychology and the University of Medicine and Dentistry of New Jersey report that quantitative EEG (QEEG) correctly identifies TBI in more than 90 percent of the cases.[26] The QEEG differs from the conventional visual EEG in that the QEEG converts the brainwaves into numerical form. Thus, the slow wave that an experienced electroencephalographer may visually identify as theta is converted to a quantitative form expressing the exact frequency, amplitude, and duration of the theta activity at any particular time during the recording. Because of the precise numerical form, the brainwave activity can be summarized and objectively analyzed for trends or for departures from average numerical values.

A number of clinical trials of neurotherapy for TBI have been reported at various clinics by neurotherapists including Jonathan Walker, a neurologist from the Southwestern Medical School in Dallas; Daniel Hoffman, a neuropsychiatrist in Englewood, Colorado; David Trudeau, formerly professor at the University of Minnesota Medical School; and psychologists Alvah Byers and Kirtley Thornton. Improvement associated with brainwave training was assessed in several ways, including computerized tests of mental abilities, self-report, and activity measures, such as successful return to work. The degree of improvement on the computerized tests of mental abilities ranged from 20 to 60 percent in the various studies.[27] Self-reports indicated improvements in the various symptoms associated with TBI of greater than 50 percent in over 80 percent of patients.[28]

Byers, whose practice is in Colorado, used neurotherapy to treat Joan, a fifty-nine-year-old woman who suffered TBI after a fall.[29] After a period of rest following her fall, Joan attempted to return to work but was eventually fired because she could not perform her tasks satisfactorily. She had problems with attention, memory, disorientation, retention of information (such as things she read), and was markedly distracted by the normal background noise of a busy office. Several other job placements all resulted in her being dismissed. She had seen many specialists, and one physician even said she was a "symptom magnifier" (a patient who exaggerates her symptoms). TBI sufferers often are told that they are malingerers, magnifiers, or just plain nuts. Byers's treatment was based on the results of an initial QEEG, which indicated regions with excessive slow-frequency amplitude and deficiencies in fast brainwave frequencies. After thirty-one sessions, Joan's self-reported severity ratings improved for twenty-one of the twenty-three rated symptoms. Her abstract reasoning measures increased by 15.4 percent, errors on a cognitive task decreased by 77.2 percent, and her estimated IQ increased by 10 percent. She could visit friends without getting lost and play cards with her granddaughter, activities she had been unable to do for six years following her accident. Given that the injury had occurred years prior to neurotherapy treatment, improvement appeared to be due to the neurotherapy intervention and not simply to recovery over time.

A good source of information on the beneficial effects of neurotherapy in the treatment of TBI, as well as other conditions, can be found on-line in the *Journal of Neurotherapy,* available on the International Society for Neurofeedback and Research website (www.ISNR.org). The bibliography on that website lists journal articles according to condition: anxiety, ADHD, depression, and so forth.

In review, neurotherapy is noninvasive; it does not zap the brain. It teaches the brain how to function efficiently. The therapy procedures are based on successful treatments that have been used for years. Therapists start by measuring the electrical activity of the brain using electrodes attached to the scalp. This electrical activity is recorded without discomfort to the client. The activity is then analyzed by looking at the different brainwaves, which provide an intimate view of the client's mental and cognitive state. The next step is devising a treatment program to create improvement. Let us turn now to the different types of brainwaves that are measured. Whether you suffer from depression or hyperactivity, the reason can be found in your brain's activity because the brain gives off an electrical signal that a neurotherapist can measure and evaluate.

CHAPTER 2

# How Do Brainwaves Work?

"Find anything in there, Doc?"

I usually reply jokingly, "I think that we can delay calling 911 for a few minutes."

Clients are understandably nervous when they are "having their head examined." Still, they know that something is not quite right for them, either mentally, cognitively, or behaviorally; otherwise, they would not be sitting in my office. "Brain examination" can be a daunting concept, and it is made more so because of the myths we have been told about the brain: "The brain has a limited capacity for recovery. You have to live with the 'cards you have been dealt.' " "Age-related changes in brain efficiency are a fact of life." "Two years after a stroke, further recovery is impossible." "Biochemical problems in the brain can be dealt with only by taking drugs."

Our growing knowledge about the brain shows clearly that these old ideas are wrong. Robert Shin of the Department of Neurology at the University of Maryland School of Medicine states, "For a long time we really didn't think the brain had [the capability to recover after injury] but now there [is] an increasing understanding that that is not true, that actually the brain can adapt, it can reorganize."[1] If you have a weak muscle in your body, exercise can increase its strength. If you have inefficiencies in brain functioning, you can exercise that function and increase its efficiency. There is ample evidence of this process. Brain imaging of blind people shows that the finger-movement and sensitivity areas in the brain expand considerably when they learn Braille.[2] Alvaro Pascual-Leone of the Neurology Department of Boston's Beth Israel Hospital also has shown that tactile (touch) sensation is processed in the visual cortex of the blind Braille reader.[3]

Edward Taub of the University of Alabama has developed a treatment for stroke patients who have only limited arm movement. In the procedure, called constraint-induced movement therapy, the unimpaired arm is temporarily restrained, and the patient is thus forced to use the impaired limb. This exercise is frustrating at first, but patients gradually gain control over their impaired limbs as they persistently attempt to perform simple tasks. Experiments on monkeys and humans have shown recovery of brain function and major changes in brain organization with this technique.[4]

Neurotherapists can usually tell clients why they have come for treatment simply by looking at their brain map. Nothing mysterious or psychic is going on. Rather, the brain signals, recorded using scalp electrodes, reveal a pattern of activity that correlates with various mental or cognitive states. Clients, having told me nothing about their condition at this point, are impressed by the accuracy of my descriptions and welcome further detailed information. The brain tells me almost everything I need to know to conduct an effective treatment program. Understanding how brainwaves work helps me identify symptoms or, in neurotherapy terms, brain inefficiencies. Such diagnostic precision gives clients confidence in the treatment and in their ability to heal or overcome their particular symptoms. They are reassured because progress can be precisely monitored during treatment. Initially concerned about having the inner workings of their brain exposed, clients rapidly become intrigued by the details of brainwave activity. The initial "Doc, do I have anything in there?" soon becomes "How did you know that, Doc?" With a pad and pen, a map of brain sites, and the raw brain data in hand, I explain brainwave activity in great detail to every client who comes to me with problems.

### Measuring Brainwave Activity

The brain produces electrical activity that can be measured with electrodes attached to the scalp. The initial reading, called the raw EEG, or raw electrical signal, is obtained from nineteen locations on the head, as shown in Figure 1. The raw signal is a composite of the various brainwaves,

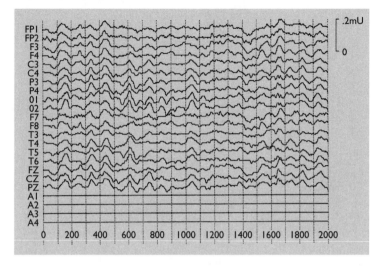

*Figure 1. Raw EEG of brainwaves from all nineteen locations.*

and the relative strength of each component wave permits accurate identification of brain inefficiencies.

In the second step of the procedure, neurotherapists examine specific locations on the head, rather than the whole brain as in the first step. Electrical activity from the brain is different depending on where it is measured. The locations used in the assessment of brainwave activity are standardized. An international system, referred to as the International 10–20 System of EEG Site Locations, defines nineteen sites for EEG assessment of the full brain map. The nineteen sites are shown in Figure 2. The locations marked A1 and A2 are the earlobes; electrodes are placed on them for electrical grounding and reference.

The brain's electrical activity is made up of wave forms varying from very slow (less than one cycle per second) to very fast (several hundred cycles per second). The activity also has long rhythms, such as changes in total strength, that vary over several hours. For research purposes neurotherapists usually specify the exact frequency and site location of any brainwaves under study. For clinical purposes, brainwaves are generally grouped into frequency bandwidths that are associated with various physical and mental states. Thus, rather than dealing with a specific frequency, such as 10 Hz, therapists assign brainwaves to bands; alpha waves, for example, which are associated with relaxed readiness, occur between

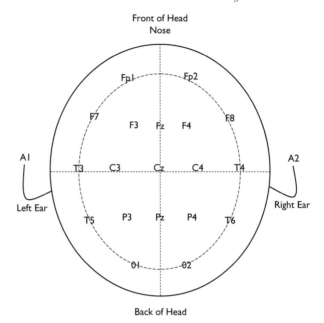

Figure 2. *International electrode site placement for EEG recording, looking down at the top of the head.*

8 and 12 Hz. Hertz (Hz) refers to cycles per second, so 10 Hz would mean a brainwave that has a frequency of 10 cycles per second. To compare this frequency to a familiar frequency, the electricity that powers your lights and small electrical appliances has a frequency of 60 Hz. The flashing red light on a bicycle for safety at night may have a frequency as low as 3 Hz.

Each of the raw electrical signals from the nineteen different brain locations, shown in Figure 1, is a composite of many different frequencies. Each recording electrode measures activity from about a hundred thousand brain cells, so the composite signal contains many different frequencies. The composite signal can be filtered to isolate activity in the six brainwave bands: delta, theta, alpha, sensory motor rhythm (SMR), beta, and high frequency (HF). The reader should keep in mind that the frequency bandwidths described here are approximations: different authors may use slightly different bandwidths for each brainwave band.

A bit of wave theory may be useful at this point. The concepts of frequency, amplitude, rhythmicity, and structure are illustrated in Figure 3. Some variations exist in the way wave characteristics are expressed by

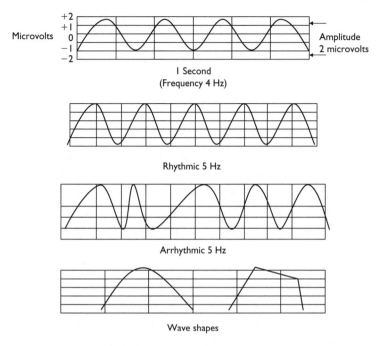

*Figure 3. Signal characteristics of brainwaves.*

different authors, but those shown in Figure 3 are common. Frequency refers to the number of cycles of the wave form that are completed each second. In the figure, the wave has four repetitions in a one-second interval, or 4 Hz. The amplitude refers to the size of the wave, measured often in microvolts (millionths of a volt). The symmetry of the wave is also important. Brainwaves are said to be synchronized, or rhythmic, when they are symmetrical. Arrhythmic, or desynchronized, brainwaves lack symmetry. A wave characteristic that is becoming increasingly important is the shape. Two examples are shown in the figure. Brainwaves that have similar frequencies but different wave shapes do not share common sources.

## Brainwave Bands

### Delta Waves

Delta activity is slow, ranging between 0.5 and 2 cycles per second (0.5–2 Hz). Associated with stages of sleep (it dominates stage 4 sleep), delta present in the EEG of an awake person has been identified with generalized brain inefficiency and with a low pain threshold. Robert Thatcher notes that at birth 40 percent of brainwave amplitude is delta as compared with less that 5 percent in the awake adult.[5] Highly rhythmic delta can be an indication of pathology, such as a traumatic brain injury.

The significance of your delta activity depends on how alert you are when the measurements are obtained. If you are drowsy, with eyes closed, high-amplitude delta waves present in the EEG indicate the early stages of sleep or drowsiness. However, if you are alert and attentive, having many delta waves may signal various types of inefficiency. High delta activity over the frontal area of the brain is often associated with chronic pain disorders such as fibromyalgia. Excessive delta activity directly on top of the head is associated with attention deficiencies and learning problems.

Too much delta activity in one area of the brain has effects quite different from those associated with excessive delta in a different area. One patient, Jim, complained of mental "fogginess" and fatigue. The brain assessment revealed several areas of inefficiency, one of which was a marked excess of delta intensity in the frontal part of the brain. Jim had Lyme disease, which, like other viral infections, can produce significant neurological symptoms caused by high frontal delta amplitude. Even after successful medical treatment of this disease, clients often express some cognitive difficulties of the kind Jim suffered from. I treated these problems by suppressing delta amplitude in the right frontal area of Jim's brain. With a visual picture of the delta activity in his brain, I helped Jim learn how to reduce the delta amplitude. Using biofeedback of the delta amplitude (a tone would signal when the amplitude was decreasing), Jim learned how to engage the mental states associated with reduced delta. After twelve sessions, Jim recovered his previous intellectual capabilities and level of vigor.

### Theta Waves

Theta is probably the most important brainwave band used in a neurotherapist's diagnosis and treatment. The significance of theta activity, between 3 and 7 Hz, is closely related to the area of the brain where the activity is measured. In most areas, theta is associated with hypoactivity (reduced activity), daydreaming, inattention, absence of directed thought, and drowsiness. A person experienced in meditation, for example, can produce many theta waves while in the meditative state. High theta amplitude is also found at times of inner focus and contemplation. In the 1970s, Elmer Green, a researcher at the Menninger Foundation in Topeka, Kansas, conducted research on the brainwave activity of psychics, healers, and mystics. In 1970, Swami Rama, a yoga master from Rishikesh, India, was "Swami in Residence" at the Menninger. In one experimental session, Swami Rama silenced his subconscious mind, and Green saw a corresponding marked increase in theta amplitude.[6] In many demonstrations, experienced meditators have markedly changed their own EEG, and healers have been able to affect the EEG of others over great distances.[7]

Theta waves are also enhanced during a hypnotic trance, and the vivid images experienced during twilight sleep are also associated with theta activity. Corydon Hammond, professor at the University of Utah School of Medicine, described some of the theta patterns associated with hypnosis and noted that the hypnotic state is characterized by an increased theta amplitude. People who are readily hypnotized show greater amplitude in the high theta (5.5 to 7.5 Hz) range than people who are not hypnotized as easily.[8] Global thinking (focusing on general ideas rather than specifics), in contrast to the logical problem solving of beta states (see below), is likewise associated with high theta activity in some areas of the brain.

Hypnotic states, twilight sleep, meditation, daydreaming—all are associated with reduced activity in the brain and the dominance of theta waves. High theta activity reflects the overall quiescence of the central nervous system. Theta activity in the back of the brain (occipital area, or occiput) is associated with the mind's ability to quiet itself. Deficient theta activity in the occiput is often associated with sleep disturbance, low stress tolerance, and predisposition to addiction. People with poor theta production in this area often cannot "shut the brain off" and suffer from anxiety-related disorders. Elevated theta amplitude is also found around the site of injuries to the brain because the injured area is not functioning at the same rate as surrounding uninjured areas.

One of my clients, Clarence, was severely agitated and looked as though he was on the verge of a breakdown. He fidgeted constantly, breathed in gasps, twitched his eyes, and made several references to his inability to cope and "go on" with life. He just could not find any peace of mind. Clarence's brain was severely deficient in theta amplitude in the occipital region. Such severe theta deficiency can be associated with many serious conditions that respond poorly to most psychoactive medications (other than heavy sedation). I pointed out to Clarence that his problems could be reduced to one cause, and that was the theta deficiency in the back of his brain. For clients with acute symptoms like Clarence, I, like many neurotherapists, adopt the "blunderbuss" approach (combining several treatments) to rapidly increase theta amplitude. After his first session, Clarence was able to get some sleep. We then embarked on a systematic neurotherapy treatment to increase and stabilize the theta brainwaves in the back of his brain. He also benefited from several psychotherapy sessions, which helped resolve some of the problems created by his severe agitation. He had developed the habit of isolating himself to deal with his severe anxiety, but after some therapy he started to socialize again. The good news from my perspective was that Clarence had the good sense to stay clean and sober. Alcohol gave him some relief, but he correctly feared that he could become dependent. He also threw away the pharmaceutical cocktails that had been prescribed by another clinician because he found that, short of sedation, they offered no relief. After thirty-one sessions over a two-and-a-half-year period, he experienced tremendous improvement.

**FREQUENTLY ASKED QUESTION**

Q: I was told to meditate to help me relax. It doesn't help, and I don't like it. Are there some people who just can't meditate?

A: Yes. People who have a deficiency of slow-frequency brainwaves in the back of the brain often can't remain still enough to meditate. Neurotherapy can create meditation-like states, and after treatment many clients are able to start a daily meditation regimen.

### Alpha Waves

Because alpha activity (8–12 Hz) is related to relaxed attentiveness, many of the first practitioners of brainwave biofeedback taught their clients to enhance their alpha waves in order to learn relaxation techniques. This narrow focus was unfortunate because it led many health care practitioners to dismiss neurotherapy as merely an esoteric form of relaxation training. Although it is true that you can become relaxed by increasing alpha waves, this use of brainwave feedback is of minor importance compared with the vast array of ways this powerful band can be used.

Alpha, in general, is the parking or idling frequency in the brain. Your brain is an enormously energy-hungry organ. It weighs only about three pounds in an adult but consumes more than 20 percent of body energy when it is working efficiently. Hence, your brain's efficiency in getting in and out of park is extremely important. The speed with which the brain's alpha waves change, an indicator of brain efficiency, can become diminished with age and with reduced mental activity. Testing alpha waves also tells us about visualization skills, visual memory, emotional trauma, and artistic skill or interest. For instance, peak performance training for athletes or for those in demanding decision-making situations is focused on amplifying the fast-frequency components of alpha waves.

Michael Doppelmayr, Wolfgang Klimesch, and their colleagues at the University of Salzburg in Austria have studied the relationship between peak alpha frequency and intellectual performance. Recall that the alpha brainwave band is between 8 and 12 Hz. These researchers have shown that the greater the amplitude of the faster alpha (over 10 Hz) relative to the slower alpha (below 10 Hz) the better one's intellectual performance.[9] Simon Hanslmayr, also at the University of Salzburg, further found that the ratio of fast to slow alpha amplitude can be increased with neurotherapy. He and his colleagues reported that such increases are directly related to improved intellectual performance.[10] These findings are consistent with the research reported by Lynda and Michael Thompson; they found that IQ scores, in general, increase by at least ten points after neurotherapy treatments.[11]

Several characteristics of alpha brainwaves are associated with cognitive efficiency. For example, slow changes in alpha amplitude between measurements made when the eyes are open and those made when the eyes are closed are frequently associated with cognitive sluggishness and memory problems. A tune-up treatment often used for elderly people who feel that they are becoming mentally sluggish or forgetful is to increase alpha parking/unparking efficiency. This type of treatment is also used to correct iatrogenic "Alzheimer's" disorder—that is, symptoms that mimic Alzheimer's but are caused by drug treatment. I frequently see elderly clients who, because they felt that they were becoming forgetful or have been told so by "concerned" others, have gone to see their physicians. The physicians, for lack of another diagnosis, tell the clients that they may be experiencing early signs of Alzheimer's disorder. These clients become upset and agitated and lose sleep, and they are often prescribed sedating medication for these problems. The effects of these medications on seniors include forgetfulness, disorientation, fatigue, and cognitive slowness—in other words, the very symptoms associated with senility. One of the great joys of my practice is seeing fearful and discouraged elderly clients gain a redefined view of themselves and their lives when I "brighten" their brains and discard the drugs. They are truly new people, with a restored sense of self-worth and robust self-confidence. Brain brightening is a simple neurotherapy procedure in which the client learns how to reduce the amount of inappropriate slow-brainwave activity, increase the frequency of the dominant alpha, and increase the rapidity of changes in alpha amplitude from eyes open to eyes closed.

**FREQUENTLY ASKED QUESTION**

Q: My psychology professor said that our brains start to decline after twenty-one years of age. I'm sure he was joking, but can neurotherapy help with old-age dementia?

A: This is one of the most rewarding applications of neurotherapy. Age-related declines can be markedly altered with brain-brightening neurotherapy. I have many clients who come in twice a year to keep their brainwaves efficient.

In one case, Julie, who appeared to be in her eighties, came in accompanied by her daughter. Both looked disheartened, and Julie looked utterly drained. She had been told that she was becoming forgetful and, as she later confided, thought that she was going to be "put away because of Alzheimer's." She wasn't sleeping well, felt sad, scared, and hopeless. I asked Julie about medications, and she said that she had recently been put on "something to calm my nerves." She also confided that she was beginning to experience the forgetfulness that others had noticed. I showed Julie where her alpha frequencies were slowing down and explained that older people often do experience slowing of the alpha brainwaves. The good news was that they could be "speeded up." I showed her an article that described the work of Thomas Budzynski on brain brightening for seniors.[12] I advised her to talk to her prescribing physician and try to discard the medications that were slowing down her alpha frequencies. The blend of eleven sessions of neurotherapy and large doses of encouragement resulted in a revitalized and happy client. Julie now comes in every three months to keep her alpha frequencies at an appropriate speed.

Just as deficiencies in alpha waves can be associated with cognitive problems, excessive alpha can be problematical as well. Too much alpha in the front of the brain can be associated with attention problems and difficulties with planning, organizing, sequencing, and following through on activities. Excessive frontal alpha can also be related to hyperverbosity (being overly talkative) and sleep disturbances. Balance of alpha frequencies in the front of the brain is also important to overall health. Richard Davidson of the Center for the Study of Emotions at the University of Wisconsin reported that when the left frontal region had much greater alpha amplitude than the right frontal region, individuals in his study were more likely to be depressed and to react more negatively to emotional situations. Infants with greater alpha amplitude in the left frontal area, in contrast to infants without this condition, were more likely to cry when separated temporarily from their mothers and had suppressed immune functioning.[13]

### Sensory Motor Rhythm

SMR is measured at sites over the top of the head from just above the tips of either ear. Beneath the skull, brain tissue in this region plays a role in touch, sensation, and movement. SMR is often considered to be in the high alpha to low beta range (13–15 Hz), which is the range that is often used to enhance peak-performance training, to brighten the brain, and to treat memory problems in elderly clients. In general, SMR is associated with body stillness and an alert mind. SMR reflects the brain's quieting of muscular tone in the body more than simply relaxation.

**CONDITIONING**

During neurotherapy the brain learns how to function efficiently in many ways. The two important ways are through operant conditioning and through classical conditioning. The basic principle of operant conditioning is that responses that are followed by pleasant or positive events are likely to be repeated and those followed by negative events occur with less frequency. When Barry Sterman wanted to teach cats to increase a particular brainwave (SMR), he structured the experimental situation so that when the rhythm increased, the cat would get a small taste of chicken broth and milk (see note 14 in this chapter). This same procedure is used today for teaching children to change a brainwave. When the brainwave moves in the desired direction, the child is rewarded with progress on a video-type game that is played only with the brain. So with Pac-Man, for example, when the brainwave is improving, Pac-Man moves across the screen and the child's game score is increased.

Classical conditioning focuses on reflexive learning by association. The usual example given is that a child learns to fear fire after being burnt. The brain-driving procedure discussed in this book is based on this principle. For example, when training the brain of a child with ADHD to reduce slow-frequency theta, the brain driver delivers a brief theta suppressing sound whenever theta is too high.

The use of SMR for clinical purposes was discovered by chance. Barry Sterman, now professor emeritus at the University of California School of Medicine, found that SMR in cats could be increased in amplitude by experimental procedures that quieted the cat's body. He further found that cats could be taught to increase the strength of SMR, and he and one of his graduate students subsequently published the first paper on the operant conditioning of brainwaves in 1968.[14] Shortly thereafter he obtained a contract from the U.S. Air Force to examine the seizures produced by rocket fuels containing hydrazine compounds. The military was concerned because of the potential danger to personnel exposed to the fuels. In the initial phase of his research, Sterman used some of the cats previously involved in SMR studies. After exposing these cats to the hydrazine compound, he observed a most curious phenomenon. Some of the cats were more resistant to seizures after being exposed to hydrazine than others. After analyzing the results, he made a remarkable discovery. Cats that had been more successful in increasing SMR strength in the previous experiment were more resistant to seizures when exposed to hydrazine.[15]

**ANIMALS IN RESEARCH**

There are horrible examples of animal abuse in research laboratories where, for often quite trivial purposes such as developing cosmetics, animals suffer greatly. The cats and rodents used in some of the research discussed in this book I am sure did experience discomfort and pain. The cases do show, however, that careful and humane research on animal subjects can have huge benefits in contributing to the reduction of human suffering. One example is the research reported in this book that was focused on finding methods for reducing the risk to people exposed to seizure-inducing aircraft fuels. This research serendipitously yielded clues to finding a treatment for drug-resistant epilepsy. I cannot speak for the cats, but I think this is an example of the benefit that can be derived from well-conceived and well-executed basic research with animals.

After this discovery, Sterman began working with human clients and successfully treated epileptic clients with neurotherapy that enhanced SMR.[16] More recently, I published my finding that neurotherapy, in addition to producing positive clinical results for epilepsy, also effectively treats "pseudo-seizure" disorders. These seizure-like episodes do not appear to be related to brain activity commonly found with seizure disorders. Pseudo-seizures include fugue states, grand mal–like thrashing, and fainting.[17]

Enhancing SMR also helps resolve many other problems related to muscular activity. The SMR procedure has been used to treat headaches, chronic pain, body tremors, dystonia, and seizure disorders that have a motor component. When I work with clients who have seizure disorders, I am aware that they may have seizures, even in my office. Seizures can take many forms, including fainting, thrashing, freezing, hypnotic-like trances, body distortions, peculiar facial tics, and trembling. A qualified and certified neurotherapist can treat these disorders by helping the client correct brainwave abnormalities that may be contributing to the problem as well as by helping the client learn to increase SMR to quiet the body.

Yana, having just learned that she was pregnant, was worried on her first visit. She had epilepsy and took antiseizure medication to control the condition. Assured by her physician that the medications were safe for pregnant women, Yana nevertheless searched the scientific literature for her own information. She found recent studies indicating that the drugs had the potential of damaging fetal development.[18] Yana also learned, through her Internet searches, that neurotherapy had been found to be effective for treating seizure disorders. Determined not to injure her unborn child, Yana started an intensive series of neurotherapy treatments. At the same time she gradually decreased her medications. Her physician, though concerned that a seizure during pregnancy could have severe effects on the fetus as well as the mother, worked with us to carefully reduce Yana's medications. Yana was also one of those fortunate people who know in advance when they are vulnerable to a seizure. Yana described this forewarning as a feeling of increased muscle tension, light-headedness, and unsteadiness. I instructed Yana to use some self-administered procedures immediately upon becoming aware of the aura that was associated with her risk of seizure. The neurotherapy treatments focused on increasing SMR and reducing slow-frequency (theta) activity. Yana reduced her medication by 50 percent after two weeks and was medication-free after her sixth week of treatment. She continued treatment on a weekly basis throughout her pregnancy and remained seizure-free. Fortunately, she had a rapid delivery without any seizures. Yana had no seizures in my office either.

**FREQUENTLY ASKED QUESTION**

Q: I am epileptic, and my doctor says I have to take medication for the rest of my life. She says there is no evidence that neurotherapy helps. Does neurotherapy reduce seizures?

A: Go to the Internet and look up neurotherapeutic treatment of epilepsy. Since the late 1960s neurotherapists have successfully treated seizure disorders.

John, however, had a full epileptic seizure on his first visit. In his late twenties, John was living with his parents because he required constant care and supervision. His condition was becoming progressively worse.

He experienced between five and twenty seizures per day, even though he was heavily medicated. I treat many clients like John. These severe chronic conditions are not going to be resolved after a few visits, but the prognosis is excellent over the long haul. John was treated twice per week for the first six months and then once per week for an additional eight months. He now receives treatment about every three weeks. His medication levels have been reduced by 75 percent, and he reports about one seizure per week.

Sterman's research is particularly good news for people with drug-refractory epilepsy. Drug-refractive patients are those who do not experience adequate seizure control with medication. The drug-refractive group constitutes a large portion of the epileptic population, and fortunately most people in this group can be treated effectively with neurotherapy. Sterman analyzed the scientific reports on neurotherapeutic treatment of epilepsy. A review of eighteen studies done at various research laboratories around the world found that 82 percent of the treated patients reported at least a 30 percent reduction in the frequency and severity of seizures, with the average reduction being over 50 percent.[19]

Brain trauma is often associated with seizure-like activity. To return to James Evans's work with violent offenders (described in Chapter 1), in which he found that most of the offenders had evidence of frontal-lobe brain damage, one hypothesis suggested by Douglas Quirk, who worked for many years in the Ontario Ministry of Correctional Services, is that dangerous offenders have had injury to brain centers associated with rage and violence.[20] There have been other reports of brain injury–related increases in inappropriate anger. Jong Kim and his associates at the Asian Medical Center in Seoul, Korea, reported that about one-third of stroke patients are unable to control anger. This anger, they report, appears to be a result of the brain injury and not simply an emotional reaction to the stroke.[21] Quirk postulated that, like Sterman's epileptic patients, violent offenders would respond favorably to SMR neurotherapy. Quirk used a testing procedure to select inmates who likely had deep brain damage. The seventy-seven selected inmates received from 0 to 120 treatments (the number of treatments being determined by factors such as paroles, transfers, and dropping out of the treatment program). Quirk reported that those violent offenders who received fewer than four treatment sessions had a recidivism rate (that is, were convicted of another violent offence within eighteen months) of 65 percent, which is the usual rate for these young male offenders. For those inmates who received more than thirty-four treatments, though, the recidivism rate was only 20 percent. Further, the recidivism rate was directly proportional to the number of treatments—the more treatments, the lower the rate. Quirk's article was published in the *Journal of Neurotherapy* shortly before his death. That article and related research can be found on the web at www. ISNR.org.

SMR neurotherapy has also successfully treated tics associated with Tourette's syndrome, a condition characterized by uncontrollable utterances and tics. Alan Strohmayer of the New York University School of Medicine reports that children who increase their SMR amplitude experience a significant reduction in tics.[22] The effects seem permanent, as reported by Raymond Daly, a psychologist at the University of Windsor in Ontario. His paper describes the successful treatment of an eleven-year-old boy who remained tic-free at a three-year follow-up session.[23] The message is clear: for people experiencing seizures, tics, or rage-related behavior, neurotherapy can make a real difference in the quality of their lives.

### Beta Waves

Beta waves cycle faster than delta, theta, alpha, and SMR, at 16–25 Hz, and are associated with processing information. When beta waves dominate, your brain is using a lot of energy, so it is important that the brain quickly ramp up to produce beta activity when required and, perhaps more important, rapidly clamp down the beta when the brain should be resting. Along with theta waves, beta activity provides critical information on the functioning of specific areas in the brain. For instance, too little beta activity in the front of the brain is associated with hypoactivity and the related problems of inattention, comprehension difficulties, and learning problems. On the flip side, too much beta power in the back of the brain can be an indicator of anxiety, low stress tolerance, sleep problems, or depression. If a client's beta activity remains high over long periods of time, during occasions when it should be diminished, the person often experiences chronic fatigue or emotional volatility. Too little beta power relative to theta waves in the central region at the top of the head is often associated with hyperactivity in children. The child's brain is understimulated in these cases, and the hyperactivity relieves the discomfort of understimulation. Drugs that stimulate the central nervous system, such as methylphenidate (Ritalin), Dexedrine, and other amphetamines, can calm the child temporarily and provide a window of opportunity during which other interventions such as neurotherapy and behavioral treatment can be undertaken. Once the children start to achieve successful results, the use of the stimulant can be slowly and progressively decreased.

## OVERLAPPING BRAINWAVE BANDS

The reader will notice that some brainwave bands overlap one another in frequencies. For example, beta can extend down into ranges lower than that discussed in this book. In this book, for beta, the bandwidth is limited to 16–25 Hz. Beta can extend down to about 12 Hz, which includes frequencies in the SMR bandwidth (13–15 Hz). Fortunately, in this case, SMR is limited to the areas over the sensory motor cortex (from ear tip to ear tip) over the top of the head. When one is recording SMR frequencies at other brain locations, the brainwave is actually beta.

There are some challenges to developing methods for distinguishing brainwaves that share overlapping frequencies. In one case, the brainwaves associated with the mirror neurons, which are implicated in imitative learning, overlap with the SMR brainwaves so neurotherapists can have difficulty separating the two different bands. Some differences are found in the shape of brainwaves from different bands that share the same frequencies. The mirror-neuron brainwaves, for example, have a jagged shape, whereas the SMR brainwaves have a smoother and more sinusoidal shape. To improve the efficacy of neurotherapy, work is progressing on developing software programs that can distinguish brainwaves based on their shape.

You can also have too much beta amplitude over most of the brain. Such excess can be the result of a brain injury, such as a stroke, or general anxiety disorders. Take Hugh, for example. He was an angry man. He had been retired for a little more than a year when he suffered a stroke. Among other complaints, he felt that fate had treated him unfairly. He had worked in a fast-paced, high-pressure occupation and had retired to the golf course. The brainwave map indicated several problem areas, some of which were the result of the stroke, but others most surely had been present prior to the incident. Hugh was deficient in theta amplitude in the back of the brain. As a result, he had poor stress tolerance and problems quieting himself. He also had excessive beta amplitude over most of the brain, a condition related to generalized anxiety. My clinical judgment was that the theta deficiency was an inherent condition predating the stroke, whereas the excessive beta amplitude was caused, or at least made worse, by the stroke.

When Hugh sat down for his brain map, he was antagonistic and red-faced. He reported that he was forgetful, became fatigued easily, and was impatient, depressed, and angry. He could not drive because he got lost easily and became extremely agitated. The map of Hugh's brainwaves certainly correlated with his behavior, and, thus, his treatment included increasing the theta amplitude in the back of the brain and reducing the beta amplitude everywhere else. Combined with the neurotherapy was some down-to-earth life-management counseling focused on breaking years of bad psychological habits: being impatient with himself and with life in general. Hugh is now back on the golf course and driving his car. He has learned to live in an essentially calm and accepting manner.

### SOME COMMON ADHD BRAINWAVE PATTERNS

| BEHAVIOR | BRAIN |
|---|---|
| Daydreams | Too much theta at the top of head |
| Is always bouncing around | Too much theta at the top of head and too much beta at the back |
| Talks too much, can't stay on an activity | Too much alpha at the front |
| Is listless, unmotivated | More beta in right front than in left front |
| Is unreasonable, defiant | More alpha in right front than in left front |
| Is slow intellectually | Too much delta in front |

### High-Frequency Waves

HF brainwaves (28–40 Hz) are measured along the middle strip of the brain, from front to back, particularly over the front part of the middle of the brain. In that location, much of the brainwave activity is thought to reflect the activity of a brain structure that lies a few centimeters below the surface. This structure, the anterior cingulate gyrus, is central to emotional functions and is also associated with obsessive and compulsive behaviors. Hammond reports that clients with obsessive-compulsive disorder (OCD) often have excessive HF amplitude over this region.[24] Detailed information about a client's OCD behaviors can be obtained by looking at the ratio of HF waves to beta waves.[25] When that ratio is large, the client usually has obsessive thought patterns. Conversely, when that ratio is low, clients are passive. Worrying and fretting are behaviors that are also often reported when high amplitudes of both beta and HF brainwaves are found along the front midline of the brain.

Therapists often find a "hot midline" in autistic children. They have a high HF-to-beta ratio, which indicates that the anterior cingulate gyrus is hyperactive. These children get stuck on themes, such as incessant repetition of a phrase, obsessive concern about an event (such as going to lunch or wanting toast for breakfast), and compulsive repetition of a behavior. Jody was an eight-year-old girl with autism, and one feature of her brainwave map was a hot midline. Once Jody got stuck on a theme, she would persist until her parents simply wore out. If you are a parent of a nonautistic

**FREQUENTLY ASKED QUESTION**

Q: My autistic daughter was treated by a nurse who conducted brainwave biofeedback. My daughter became much worse. The nurse said that this outcome had nothing to do with her treatment and that my child was not a good candidate for neurotherapy. Did neurotherapy make my child worse?

A: Possibly, particularly if the treatment was "one size fits all." In some cases of autism, a certain area of the brain must be kept calm during early treatment or the condition can markedly worsen. "One size fits all" treatments aren't precise enough for such conditions. Precision treatment is based on a careful assessment and involves correcting the brain inefficiencies while monitoring other areas of the brain to minimize any temporary worsening of specific autistic symptoms. Clearly, only certified and licensed professionals with the capability to do full brain assessments are qualified to treat such cases.

child, you may think that your child too has this skill of persisting until you
finally give in. Multiply this common stubbornness by a factor of twenty,
and you have an idea of Jody's behavior. This sort of obsessiveness interferes
with the child's progress in neurotherapy, so we usually treat this area of the
brain first. Jody required nine sessions to suppress the HF brainwave amplitude to the point where she could let go of her obsessive themes during
treatment.


**Frequency: Forty Hz**


In addition to brainwave bands, several specific frequencies are important in neurotherapy; 40 Hz is one of them. This frequency has been
found to be associated with sharp focus, language comprehension, feelings of enhanced personal insight, memory retention, and learning.
Some children with learning disorders do not show any 40-Hz increase
when intellectually challenged. Hypnotherapists have reported a spike
of 40-Hz activity during some important phases of hypnosis, and many
neurotherapists engaged in peak-performance training use 40-Hz
enhancement to create sharp focus and feelings of being energized, creative, and insightful. The 40-Hz activity is found throughout the brain.
For this reason, 40-Hz enhancement training generally helps the various
parts of the brain work together; when they do, learning, creativity, disciplined focus, and cognitive energy are increased. The 40-Hz activity
appears to be associated with recruiting various areas of the brain to take
in information. It optimizes the integration and transfer of information.
Such training can help considerably when the client is having difficulty
with retention and retrieval of information.

    As discussed previously, clients interested in optimizing their cognitive
function often receive neurotherapy on an ongoing basis. Certainly, for
seniors, optimal-functioning training mitigates non-Alzheimer's dementias and delays the onset of Alzheimer's. For clients not yet experiencing
age-related declines, optimal-functioning training increases cognitive efficiency. Many executives and athletes choose to train the brain on a systematic schedule, just as one might routinely go to a gym to exercise your
body. After a brain assessment and the correction of any anomalies, training focuses on optimizing the alpha brainwaves and increasing the amplitude

of 40-Hz activity. Often increasing 40-Hz activity is done while the client is engaged in a cognitive task such as reading. Optimal-performance clients drop in every month or so and, like Marlene, may also come in and say, "Tune me up, Doc; I have a critical meeting this afternoon." Treating clients in order to improve functioning in this way is clearly less worrisome than treating clients with pathologies.

In the next chapter we turn our attention to the details of interpreting the activity of the brain. The purpose of brain mapping is to determine the areas of the brain that are not functioning efficiently. These inefficiencies are directly related to the symptoms or complaints that clients want corrected. As we will see, brainwaves reflect behavior differently depending on the brain location. Knowing how the geography of the brain works can help therapists find ways to improve functioning.

CHAPTER 3

## Interpreting the Signals of the Brain

How does a neurotherapist interpret brainwave activity? What does the brain activity of a "normal" brain look like? Scientists have made efforts to determine "normal" brain maps. "Normal" folks are those whose psychological assessments and self-reports do not reveal any disorders. Interestingly, the percentage of individuals who test "normal" on psychological tests is only about 40 percent. Thus, the "normal" population is in the minority, not the majority. Most of us have problems!

From a clinical perspective, the concept of "normal" is not useful. Clients do not come to neurotherapists and say, "Find something in my brain that is not normal." Rather, they say they cannot sleep, are depressed or forgetful, or cannot pay attention. In fact, I usually do not encourage clients to tell me much about their problems. I let the initial brain assessment tell me. After that I can tell clients the reasons they are now sitting in my office with what clients state is remarkable accuracy. Potentially, the brainwave patterns tell us nearly everything we need to know. The task for the neurotherapist is to learn how to decipher and find meaning in the patterns of the brain activity that are measured.

In the early years of my practice, I carried out psychological testing on all clients. I measured various psychological profiles and physical symptoms, asked for life stories, and the like. However, the results of this laborious and costly process had virtually no bearing on my therapeutic decisions. The brain map corroborated the client's clinical history, and I found myself relying increasingly on the brain map alone to direct how the patient's therapy would go. Today the clinical portrait that I obtain on a client is brief, consisting essentially of the history of any medications, neurological symptoms, seizures, or head injuries. If clients proceed to elaborate on their problems, I usually ask them to wait until after I do the brain map for, more often than not, I can give them a precise description of their problems based on the brain map alone. One challenge I enjoy occurs when a parent states that she is not going to let me test her child until I test her first. If my assessment of her condition is accurate, then she will bring her child to see me. After many years of practice, with these situations occurring several times each month, I still have a 100 percent success rate with respect to convincing mothers that a brain map gives an impressive amount of information and is worth doing with their children. This result speaks to the remarkable accuracy of brain assessments. After interpreting the brain map, I then ask the client to provide additional relevant data, which might include social and emotional events that could have a bearing on how the therapy should proceed.

As an example, I had a woman who complained of severe sleep disturbances. I obtained a brief history of her medications, the duration of the disorder, and asked whether she had ever had a head injury, severe illness, or seizures. I determined the areas in the brain that related to the disturbances. As is often found, this client had a deficiency of theta amplitude in the back of her brain and a mild elevation of alpha amplitude in the front part of her brain. These two conditions are quite common with clients who complain of sleep disturbances. However, she also showed the brainwave pattern associated with emotional trauma. I reviewed the results of her brain map and then obtained some additional information, particularly regarding the potential source of the trauma. I found during the follow-up questioning that this client had once been attacked when she was asleep and then raped. Clearly in such a case, adjusting the brain imbalance is only part of the therapy. The other component is the psychological part of the term *psychoneurophysiology*.

Assessing five specific sites identifies the neurological bases for most of the problems reported by clients. My descriptions of these five brain regions in this chapter provide general guidelines for identifying problem areas. Many psychological conditions are revealed in *brain signatures*, which are patterns in brain activity that can be readily identified.

A brain map must include the following five locations: the occiput, or back of the brain; the area over the sensory motor cortex, or top of the head; and three locations over the frontal cortex, or front of the brain. Once we have a firm understanding of the information these sites provide, we can look at brainwave data recorded from both child and adult clients that cover a wide range of clinical problems.

## Occiput

One of the most critical brain areas is a site at the back of the brain, labeled O1 in Figure 2 (Chapter 2). In this area of the brain, neurotherapists look for several indicators of healthy brain functioning.

### *Theta and Beta Disturbances*

If you are relaxed and your eyes are open, the theta/beta ratio should be around two to one—that is, the amplitude of the theta (3–7 Hz) brainwaves should be twice that of the beta (16–25 Hz) waves. This ratio is typically a bit higher in young children and a bit lower in adults, but a value of two is a good guideline. Theta activity in the back of the brain indicates the brain's ability to quiet itself. When the ratio of the amplitude of the theta to beta waves falls much below two, agitation in the central nervous system is common. In other words, clients find it difficult to shut off the brain. They often experience nonspecific anxiety and have a low tolerance for stress.

In extreme cases, this level of agitation leads to a predisposition to addictive behavior. The addiction can be to almost anything: alcohol, nonmedical drugs, prescription medications, food, sex, gambling, exercise, television, a person, or other calming or distracting situations. One subtype of genetically predisposed alcoholism is characterized by slow-brainwave deficiencies in the back of the brain; nondrinking young male children of fathers with this type of alcoholism often show this same deficiency of theta waves. An inherited predisposition toward alcohol abuse and addiction has been established both in animal and in human studies. Marc Schuckit, presently a professor at the University of California, San Francisco, studied children of alcoholics and found that they were three times more likely to become alcoholics than children of nonalcoholic parents.[1] This effect could, theoretically, be cultural and not genetic, but studies of adopted children and twins have established a genetic component to these addictive disorders.

The Collaborative Study of the Genetics of Alcoholism is a large collaborative research project being undertaken at many medical centers and universities. This study involves mapping human DNA to determine the genetic predisposition to alcoholism. The data from this study are suggesting that the susceptibility to alcoholism is likely linked to several genes. The genes can have both a predisposing as well as a protective effect; one does not inherit a disease of alcoholism but rather a predisposition to alcoholism. Alcoholism is thus a combination of genetic predisposition and environmental causes, and it is likely that there are many subtypes of alcoholism depending on the genetic predisposition, including subtypes that are linked primarily to environmental conditions and not to genetic predispositions. The genetic predispositions are associated with brainwave differences.[2]

**FREQUENTLY ASKED QUESTION**

Q: I come from a long line of alcoholics, so obviously it's genetic. Can neurotherapy help my predisposition toward alcoholism?

A: The brain is remarkably plastic, meaning it can be modified. So even genetic conditions can be modified.

The hyperactivity of some children seems to stem from this same deficiency of slow-wave amplitude in the back of the brain. They cannot quiet themselves. They are fidgety and are profoundly uncomfortable when inactive. The adult with this deficiency consumes alcohol because it feels good. The alcohol provides an increase in slow-wave activity or a decrease in beta activity in the back of the brain. People with this condition are self-medicating to compensate for the deficiency in theta activity or, more generally, for the brain's inability to calm the central nervous system.

This deficiency is also related to anxiety disorders. Clients with marked deficiencies always complain of chronic anxiety. However, because not all clients with severe anxiety have this deficiency, neurotherapists cannot use the same treatment for all anxious clients. E. Roy John, director of the Brain Research Laboratories at the New York

University Medical Center, points out that an array of different brain-wave profiles are associated with anxiety disorders.[3] Although a deficiency of theta waves in the back of the brain is a prominent high-anxiety brain signature, some anxiety profiles show excess alpha in the front of the brain or over much of the cortex. Some of these patterns are specifically associated with different types of anxiety—for example, anxiety that is the result of a specific traumatic event, such as a serious illness, or generalized, chronic anxiety. Blair Simpson from the Department of Psychiatry at Columbia University Medical School found that alpha waves can shift in response to a specific threat.[4] When patients with OCD are confronted with items that provoke their symptoms, alpha power shifts from the front of the brain to the back. These differences underline the fact that an initial brainwave assessment is essential to determine the exact location and nature of the brainwave abnormalities.

Related conditions that neurotherapists see with increasing frequency are syndromes associated with prescription-drug withdrawal—for example, symptoms that occur when a benzodiazepine such as Valium is discontinued. These clients usually have a long history of drug use and complain of severe anxiety and sleep problems. The damaging effects of the long-term use of these drugs cannot be underestimated. Benzodiazepine withdrawal can last from a few days to many months and occasionally years. Heather Ashton, professor in the Division of Psychiatry at the University of Newcastle in England, has found that these drugs often cause anxiety and serious sensory and motor problems. She points out that benzodiazepines may cause not only slowly reversible changes in the brain but also some damage to the brain neurons.[5] These clients generally have an extremely low theta/beta ratio, and the treatment for this condition, like that for some forms of genetic alcoholism, is to increase theta amplitude or decrease beta amplitude (or both) in the occiput of the brain. Whether the low-amplitude theta activity is a consequence of drug use or reflects the condition for which the drug was prescribed is debatable, but making this determination is not important for treating the condition. One intervenes to normalize the EEG, regardless of the cause of the pattern.

In the initial brain-mapping assessment, after thirty seconds of eyes-open recording, clients close their eyes for fifteen seconds and then open them again for an additional fifteen seconds. When the eyes are closed, the therapist should see either no change or an increase in the theta/beta ratio. Because the brain has no visual processing to do when the eyes are closed, the occipital region, where some key aspects of visual processing take place, can rest, as indicated by increased alpha in particular. If the theta/beta ratio drops 20 percent or more when the eyes are closed, sleep disturbances are suspected. These clients often complain of trouble getting to sleep (although they may also complain of wakening and then being unable to regain sleep) or of restless sleep that leaves them still exhausted even after many hours. If the theta/beta ratio is low in the eyes-open condition, then even though there is no further drop in the ratio, sleep problems are often apparent. The low theta/beta ratio should be corrected regardless. If clients are alcoholics, they may not be aware of sleep problems because of the self-medicating use of alcohol.

Excessively high theta amplitude in the back portions of the brain is often found in children with autism and Asperger's and in children with intellectual challenges. The high-amplitude slow-frequency brainwaves in the back areas of the brain have likewise been observed by Michael and Lynda Thompson of the ADD Centre in Toronto, leaders in the development of neurofeedback treatments for children with these conditions.[6] High theta/beta ratios over diffuse brain areas usually indicate compromised brain functioning. These high ratios in the back of the brain are related to the detached states seen in autism; the children appear to be in a different world, out of touch with the events going on around them.

### Alpha Response

The other important brainwave band to consider at the occiput is alpha. When the client goes from eyes open to eyes closed to eyes open again, the neurotherapist should observe a large increase in the alpha amplitude during the eyes-closed phase. In the back of the brain, the jump up should be at least 50 percent from eyes open to eyes closed. Further, the alpha amplitude should return to the first eyes-open level within a few seconds of reopening the eyes.

If the increase in alpha amplitude is low, the person often has problems seeing things spatially. For example, a metalwork artist who had a deficient alpha response resulting from a recent emotional trauma reported that she had difficulty visualizing what she wanted to construct. She found that visualization came slowly and with considerable fatigue, a condition that started only after she had experienced the trauma. In such cases, the neurotherapist also needs to look at the alpha response in other areas of the brain to determine whether there is a generalized alpha deficiency.

If the alpha level drops from the eyes-open to the eyes-closed phase, the client may have been exposed to traumatic stress or may be anticipating a life-threatening or severely traumatic event. This possibility is particularly likely if the decrease in eyes-closed alpha amplitude is also found on top of the brain. I discovered this relationship between a negative alpha response (a decrease in alpha amplitude with eyes closed) and traumatic stress when I treated Vietnam combat veterans diagnosed with PTSD. These clients suffer from severe flashbacks, a realistic reexperiencing of the traumatic event in all its vividness. They are thrust back into the trauma emotionally, visually, and aurally, and all show a negative alpha response. If we ponder this response for a moment, we can see the brain's wisdom. Increased alpha amplitude with eyes closed indicates a capability for visualization. Hence, the brain is protecting itself by suppressing the alpha response, thereby limiting the possibility of visualizing the nightmarish experiences.

Vulnerability to PTSD has a genetic component. All people exposed to the same traumatic circumstances do not develop PTSD. Genetic vulnerability to developing the symptoms of PTSD appears to depend on the type of assault. As reported by Murray Stein of the Department of Psychiatry at the University of California at San Diego, studies of identical and fraternal twins showed that for trauma caused by assault (such as robbery or sexual assault) genetic predisposition was a factor. However, for trauma not involving an assault (such as auto accidents) genetic predisposition was not a factor.[7]

The negative alpha response also occurs in other clients who have been traumatized or are facing potential life-threatening situations. For instance, several clients scheduled for aggressive surgery for the treatment of cancer have shown this deficiency. Likewise, some women admitted to being raped or being the victims of incest when I first discussed the negative alpha response with them. When this negative alpha signature is observed in children, a full probe of a history of potential trauma is indicated.

Often parents are initially unaware of the importance of a traumatic event involving their children. In one case, a child who showed this alpha deficiency had experienced an injury of the upper mouth. The injury had occurred a few weeks before the assessment, and the parents did not associate this episode with the traumatic stress I described to them. After speaking with the child, though, I realized how traumatic the event was for her. The injury had required emergency hospital treatment. In addition, she had watched a TV program shortly before her injury that portrayed, in her mind, a similar situation, only in that case the child had died. She thought she was experiencing a life-threatening situation when she was injured and later rushed to the emergency room. The event registered weeks later in the brainwave signature characterized by the low-level alpha response.

Another case involved a boy who was being assessed for ADD-like symptoms. The brain map showed the trauma signature, but the parents initially couldn't remember any traumatic events. After some thought it occurred to one of them that the child had been traumatized by two badly handled surgical procedures. He had required genital surgery, which was first attempted around the age of two years. He was taken from the parents by hospital staff, was restrained while being given an anaesthetic, and then underwent surgery. The surgery was unsuccessful and had to be repeated two years later. The second episode was even more traumatic than the first. The child, again deprived of parental comfort and support, was strapped, hysterically screaming, to a gurney. He was then brought into what must have been a terrifying place, the surgical arena, and anesthetised. In addition to the neurotherapy, this child received some therapy with his family that successfully resolved some of the issues related to the trauma as well as restoring a robust alpha response.

**FREQUENTLY ASKED QUESTION**

Q: My son uses drugs. He won't come to see you, and I think the reason is because he thinks you will be able to tell that he has used drugs. Can you tell from his brain if he has used drugs?

A: We can see specific patterns in some brainwaves associated with certain drugs. But the drug itself may increase the brainwave that I am trying to strengthen with neurotherapy, thus masking underlying brainwave abnormalities and minimizing the effectiveness of the treatment. I explain this problem to the addict-client, and we work out a deal about staying clean for a number of hours before treatment.

The rate of decrease in alpha waves also matters. When the eyes are again opened, the alpha amplitude should drop back to the previous eyes-open level within a few seconds. Delayed alpha decrease is often found in conditions of cognitive sluggishness, a frequent complaint of elderly clients. As discussed in Chapter 2, alpha brainwaves can be thought of as the parking or resting condition for the neurons in the brain. Rapid movement in and out of the states of rest and activity is important for brain efficiency. Rapid alpha enhancement and blocking are also important in decision making. To continue with the parking or resting metaphor, rapidly changing from the resting state to the active state should facilitate information processing. As mentioned in Chapter 2, peak-performance training usually includes training in rapid alpha changes.

What about large alpha enhancement? I recognized this interesting phenomenon after assessing many hundreds of children and adults. An increase in alpha amplitude with eyes closed of 300 percent or more often reveals artistic talent or interest. I have labeled this large alpha increase the *artist signature,* as noted in Chapter 1 with Jason. When I observe this marked amplitude enhancement, I offer the speculation that the client likes activities that require visualization, such as art, dance, or model making. Usually, I receive an affirmative response from the client or parents. This can be an extraordinary esteem booster for children who have a negative view of their intellectual merits because of an attention deficiency.

In the eyes-open condition, when neurotherapists see large alpha amplitudes in adults, they probe to determine whether the client has a history of cocaine or marijuana use. Many EEG studies have shown that long-time use or withdrawal from cocaine and cannabis is associated with excessive high-amplitude alpha activity over much of the brain, including the occiput. Psychologist Leslie Prichep and colleagues at the Department of Psychiatry at the New York University School of Medicine have reported that not only do crack-cocaine users show elevated alpha amplitude, but toddlers who have been exposed to the substance in the uterus show EEG patterns remarkably similar to those of their substance-abusing mothers.[8] Thus, although high-amplitude alpha may indicate an artistic skill, it may also indicate problems with drugs. The discriminating factor is usually that drug-enhanced alpha is more diffuse and apparent in both eyes-open and eyes-closed conditions, whereas artistic high alpha is most prominent from the center to the back of the brain under eyes-closed conditions.

In sum, we can gain an enormous amount of useful data from the back of the brain. The information not only validates the client's complaints but also specifies exact conditions for treatment. All this valuable information is obtained in a mere sixty seconds of brainwave recording.

## Sensory Motor Cortex

The next site (labeled Cz in Figure 2 in Chapter 2) considered in the assessment is located at the top of the brain. The sensory motor cortex, as the name implies, is a central location for sensory and motor functioning. As shown in Figure 4, specific parts of the brain control different parts of our bodies and thought processes. The sensory motor cortex plays an important role in the diagnosis and treatment of learning, attention, and memory problems. This site is frequently used in treatment for both historical and pragmatic reasons. At the center of the brain, it was an obvious choice of early investigators simply because of its location.

Measurements at Cz provide a general view of activity in a wide area that spreads over both sides of the brain and forward to the frontal lobes. This location was so significant that many early therapists restricted their efforts to it alone because they believed that it reflected many

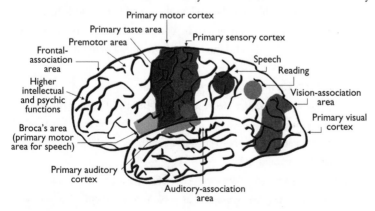

*Figure 4. The sensory motor cortex. Note the locations of the areas for both movement and sensation.*

other brain centers. It is also less prone to artifact than other sites because it is furthest from the jaws (which produce muscle artifact and thus increase the amplitude of fast frequencies such as SMR and beta) and not too close to the eyes (which produce slow-wave artifact, which increases delta and theta amplitude).

The assessment at the top of the brain requires recording approximately 150 seconds of good data. Assessments are made during both eyes-open and eyes-closed conditions and during a cognitive challenge such as reading or doing mental arithmetic. As was the case at the back of the brain, the theta/beta ratio here is of major importance, but with a key difference. At the occiput the therapist wants the theta/beta ratio to be high, over two or so, whereas at the top the ratio should be low, below two. Again, young children show higher theta/beta ratios than adults, a fact that reflects the developmental stages of the child. Children have higher theta amplitudes than adults, so an average theta/beta ratio of, say, 2.5 with a child does not raise the same concerns as it does with a forty-year-old adult.

When the eyes are open and the theta/beta ratio is much above two, we suspect attention problems. This suspicion is further clarified by a cognitive challenge. Let's say a child has an at-rest, eyes-open theta/beta ratio of 2.5, but when performing some mental activity such as reading, the ratio drops to 1.7. In this case, there is likely to be little problem with attention. The child may be prone to a bit more daydreaming than other children of a similar age, but the brain can focus when challenged. If the theta/beta ratio remains high under both at-rest and challenge conditions, then attention difficulties are probable. Further, when the theta/beta ratio is high under challenge, comprehension may also be compromised. The brain simply is not active enough for the child to retain the material being read.

**FREQUENTLY ASKED QUESTION**

Q: My husband thinks that neurotherapy is "BS" because our daughter's brainwave ratios became worse after we started treatment, even though her teacher felt she was improving. Is the treatment working even though the numbers got worse?

A: Successfully treated children with ADD often show brainwave ratios that seem to be shifting the wrong direction early in treatment. After several neurotherapy sessions, these ratios start to move in a positive direction.

A far more serious problem occurs with large increases in the theta/beta ratio during a cognitive challenge. For example, if a ten-year-old boy has a theta/beta ratio of 2.0 with eyes open at rest, but that ratio jumps to 2.6 when he does mental arithmetic, the child usually has an attention problem. This pattern is quite common, particularly in male children. The theta/beta ratio looks fine when the brain is at rest. However, when challenged, the brain, as I frequently say, "goes the wrong way." Even though the child is trying to concentrate, the brain produces a wave form associated with daydreaming. This is an extremely frustrating condition for the child. The harder he tries, the worse the attention problem becomes. If he is told that he is not trying, the child often simply gives up. When the theta/beta ratio goes up after reading or remains at a high level after the task is completed, we then suspect a problem with retention. When I see this pattern, I ask the client, "Do you frequently find that after reading a paragraph or page of a book, you can't remember what you have just read?" The answer invariably is yes.

The change in alpha-band activity between eyes-open and eyes-closed conditions is an important diagnostic indicator, as mentioned in the previous section. The increase in alpha amplitude when the eyes are closed (called the alpha response) should be rapid, within a second, as indicated by a jump on the computer monitor. The change should be at least 30 percent, such as a change from 10 microvolts to 13 microvolts when the eyes are closed. A low increase or a decrease can have several meanings. An alpha response that is deficient at the top of the brain but not at the occiput can indicate poor short-term visual memory. This can be a serious problem with reading or mathematics, for example, which are visually-based activities. Individuals with this limited alpha response often do not read novels for pleasure because reading a novel is rather like playing a movie in your head, and this visual script does not run smoothly for them. In other words, when the alpha response is limited, the associated visualization skills may be limited. I often ask a person with a limited alpha response how she remembers numbers she looks up in the phone book before making a telephone call. "If the phonebook is at one side of the room but the telephone is on the other side, can you remember the number after you cross the room to the telephone?" The answer is usually no.

If the alpha response is absent in both brain locations, then a history of trauma is likely. This history can be associated with many psychological as well as cognitive/learning difficulties. The good news is that these difficulties can usually be readily addressed neurotherapeutically. But, for complete healing, psychotherapy is necessary as well. The neurotherapeutic treatment may precipitate a rush of emotion-triggering memories that have been repressed for a long time. Flashbacks and other trauma-related episodes during treatment are not uncommon. The neurotherapist must have the psychological skills to guide the client during these emotionally important phases of the treatment. If the neurotherapist is not qualified in this regard, arrangements for the client to work with a qualified psychotherapist are essential. Clients may not even be aware of any trauma, although in my experience they always admit to no recall or confusing recall of certain periods in their past. This response can come from victims of abuse who have deeply repressed memories of the traumatic event.

Sometimes these emotional episodes are resolved rapidly with minimal distress. Clients report increased recall of dreams, often with psychologically intriguing content. They also frequently comment that they are experiencing increased recall of past events, often with interesting sensory memories such as odors and old melodies. It seems as though the client is involved in self-directed psychotherapy structured by dream content and memories that have been evoked by the neurotherapy. In simple terms, my observations of these clients strongly suggest that by releasing the alpha response and increasing theta amplitude, neurotherapy opens the emotional memory banks and, at the same time, strengthens the mind's natural self-healing. Some clients need outside help, whereas others progress well with neurotherapy alone. In general, neurotherapists trained in psychotherapy do some psychotherapy in every session.

**FREQUENTLY ASKED QUESTION**

Q: I had an alpha/theta treatment at the back of my head, and that night I had many dreams. The next day I was quite emotional but after a few days I felt great. What happened?

A: Clients frequently recall long-forgotten events, often from childhood. Some of these memories can be sad or even traumatic as well as happy. You have experienced a psychological processing of those long-forgotten events.

Margaret was an attractive woman who reminded me of a wounded dog. Her face muscles were flaccid and droopy. She seemed so terribly sad. Her appearance was also unkempt. Nothing matched, and her clothes were all drab. Margaret seemed too tired to cry. She sat forward in her chair, and, without emotion, she said that she was worn out and depressed and that life offered nothing for her. Margaret's brain map showed several areas of abnormality, one of which was the trauma signature. I asked her if she had ever been traumatized. She said that her grandfather had been abusive. She remembered being hit, shouted at, and "touched the wrong way." She said she had no recall of any sexual activity other than touching. When the slow-frequency amplitude was eventually released, Margaret had a major emotional reaction. A memory of sexual abuse by her grandfather and her brothers came flooding back to her. Her eyes widened and she started gasping. Tears started pouring down her cheeks and she moaned "Oh no!" over and over again. Many clients yell or scream during these emotional episodes, but Margaret just sobbed and moaned. Resolving the emotional trauma required psychotherapy as well as neurotherapy, with a positive result. Therapists often comment that you can assess therapeutic progress by a client's appearance. This was certainly the case with Margaret. She started dressing with care, and her facial muscles gained good tone.

Another factor that must be considered when correcting slow-wave deficiencies at these two brain sites is the "false-memory syndrome." A serious therapeutic, legal, and family-dynamic issue, the false-memory syndrome refers to inaccurately remembering past episodes. These episodes, usually traumatic, are repressed and then revealed after therapeutic intervention. However, the memories are not real but rather are the product of childhood dreams or fantasy states, current attitudes and expectations, or fuzzy traces of actual events.

Charles Brainerd, a professor at the University of Arizona, has studied false memories in children.[9] They result from incorporating false information into memories of actual events. A person may recall having gone to an amusement park as a child and having ridden on a Ferris wheel. The memory of going to an amusement park may be accurate, but the memory of riding on a Ferris wheel may be false. Riding on the Ferris wheel is consistent with having spent time in the amusement park but, in this case, is nonetheless not true. Brainerd's work has shown that the vulnerability to false memories is higher in children than in adults and that the vulnerability in children varies with age. Younger children may be less vulnerable than adolescent children.

These constructed memories can be so vivid that the client is convinced they really happened. Further, unskilled therapists often inadvertently facilitate the false-memory process because they expect to find early childhood trauma. Hypnotherapists frequently encounter this sort of problem. The critical events, uncovered during hypnosis, can be extremely problematical, and validation of the recovered "memories" can be difficult if not impossible. Neurotherapists can face similar problems because slow-brainwave enhancement often mimics the effects of hypnosis. Dealing with memories, both valid and false, that are emotionally important to a client requires a thoroughly experienced psychotherapist.

In an interesting example of the false-memory problem, Nancy was convinced that she had been physically abused by her father as a young child. She remembered being severely frightened, being unable to breathe with her heart pounding, and feeling a marked premonition of death. After extensive probing it appeared likely that her memories were of panic attacks. Nancy had, in fact, suffered from panic disorder until recently, when she was successfully treated for the condition. Nancy's memory of having been physically hurt by her father could be an example of Brainerd's theory. Nancy's childhood panic attacks appeared to have been real, as was her fear of her threatening father. Her vague recall of her father actually striking her, even if untrue, was consistent with her emotional memory.

Another example involved Sandra, a woman in her twenties who was convinced she had been sexually abused by her father. Sandra had no memory of these events, but she maintained that the psychological problems she had could have been caused only by early sexual abuse, the memories of which she had subsequently repressed. Moreover, she had already accused her father of sexual abuse, and these accusations were causing a family crisis. Although Sandra came to me for the treatment of specific symptoms, I immediately realized that she expected me to verify her assumption about sexual abuse. I told her that I could not do so. I could, however, treat her symptoms provided her commitment was to treatment and not to justifying her actions against her father. Sandra stayed in treatment with me for a short while, but then moved on to a therapist who "specialized" in the treatment of women with sexual-abuse histories. She returned to treatment with me after a year or so. She had come to the conclusion that she needed to address her problems rather than continue in her attempts to recall sexual abuse. Sandra is in good shape now, after eighteen months in treatment. Even during emotional episodes she never recalled any incidents of her father's sexually abusing her.

Sandra was a victim of a fad in the clinical treatment of women with chronic stress. A wave of therapists claimed that certain symptoms were caused unequivocally by childhood sexual abuse, and even though the theory was shown to be false, tragically some families were ruined. Tamara Sbraga, a professor at Central Michigan University, and William O'Donohue from the University of Nevada published a review of this problem in 2003.[10] These authors report that 15 percent of male and 25 percent of female children have experienced sexual abuse. But they point out that there is no evidence of any symptom markers of childhood sexual abuse. They strongly advise mental-health professionals not to provide opinions on whether a client was sexually abused as a child based only on symptoms.

**FREQUENTLY ASKED QUESTION**

Q: I have heard that many professional athletes have been treated by neurotherapists. Can neurotherapy improve the performance of activities other than sports?

A: Very decidedly so. At the very least, neurotherapy will increase your IQ.

As at the occiput, the average peak frequency of the alpha band at the top of the brain is important. Peak frequency refers to the brainwave frequency that has, on average, the highest electrical amplitude. Alpha peak frequency is directly associated with cognitive efficiency. Research at the University of Salzburg in Austria by Wolfgang Klimesch, Michael Doppelmayr, and their associates has shown that increasing the amplitude of the faster alpha frequencies results in improved intellectual performance.[11] Diagnostically, neurotherapists look for either a slow peak alpha frequency (under 9.5 Hz) or a high ratio of slow alpha (8 to 9 Hz) to fast alpha (11 to 12 Hz).

Activity in adults that is less than 9.5 Hz, on average, can be related to mental sluggishness. Slow alpha has also been associated with Alzheimer's as well as with other dementias. Lynda and Michael Thompson point to a diffuse increase in slow-wave amplitude (that is, slow alpha and theta) and a slowing of peak frequency of alpha with these dementia conditions. Further, they report, the slowing of alpha is proportional to the severity of the dementia.[12] James Evans, a professor at the University of South Carolina, and his associates compared the peak alpha frequency of children with precocious reading ability with that of age-level readers. He reports that, on average, the precocious readers' peak alpha frequency was about 5.2 percent faster than that of the grade-level readers.[13]

At the top of the brain, the alpha response should occur rapidly when the eyes close and should drop rapidly when the eyes are again opened. A sluggish alpha response can reflect cognitive "fogginess," such as the "fibro-fog" that many clients with fibromyalgia complain about.

The summated amplitude ($\Sigma A$) of brain activity is the total sum of the average electrical amplitude of the theta, alpha, and beta bandwidths. Brainwave amplitude can vary over the course of a day and can be affected by the use of drugs, physical health, the thickness of the skull, and other factors. Regardless of the time of day and physical condition, one should find the $\Sigma A$ to be in the range of 25–60 microvolts (in general, children have higher amplitudes than adults). Much higher summated amplitudes often mean that parts of the brain are not working together. The brain is a vast system of specialized units that have many complex interactions. These units are not truly independent but rather have many reciprocal connections with other centers in the brain. High summated amplitudes indicate that the connections among different brain centers are compromised. The brain is functioning in a "stuck" manner. This profile is often found in children who are developmentally "stuck," autistic, or intellectually challenged. Ironically, those children who have serious problems with intellectual strengths have brain maps that reveal enormous energy output from the brain, energy that is not harnessed properly. High summated amplitude is also frequently found in brain maps of clients with TBI, such as a head injury from an automobile accident. Such elevations are also frequently observed in clients who have suffered strokes.

The various motor and sensory functions for different body areas are located at specific locations on the sensory motor cortex. For diagnostic purposes, we measure brainwaves at this location to assess cognitive and emotional functions. Some forms of ADD are found to be associated with excessive theta amplitude in this region, and the seizure threshold for epileptics likewise is found to be related to the ratio of the amplitudes of theta and SMR. Inefficiencies in short-term memory can be assessed by looking at the strength of the alpha changes, and these same brainwaves can be an indicator of serious emotional trauma. Stroke and head-injured clients who experience body-movement problems also show brainwave irregularities in this region.

## Frontal Lobes and Frontal Midline

The frontal lobes (F3 is the left lobe and F4 is the right lobe in Figure 2 in Chapter 2) are the executive portions of the brain. Consider them to be your mental managers. Traditionally, the left lobe is thought to control the rational, objective, quantified, and linear activities of the brain. The right lobe controls the emotional, subjective, creative, parallel, and associative brain functions.

Frontal-lobe dysfunctions can have severe behavioral and emotional effects. Recall the case of Vincent in Chapter 2; an injury to the right frontal lobe resulted in his having impulse and anger-control problems. Ricardo Weinstein did brainwave assessments of twenty death-row inmates and found that all had clear evidence of frontal-lobe dysfunction; this finding indicates the critical importance of this area of the brain.[14] Interpreting brain activity in the frontal lobes is complicated, and a neurotherapist must be cautious when examining brainwave patterns and looking for a characteristic or symptom that matches the brainwave profile.

Once again, the ratio of theta to beta brainwaves is a highly important measure at the frontal-lobe locations. If the theta/beta ratio is higher in the left frontal lobe than in the right, the neurotherapist will probe the client for depressed mood states. However, some learning disabilities, such as dyslexia, are often associated with a high theta/beta ratio in the left frontal lobe. Another indicator of depression is the right/left beta/beta ratio. If beta activity at the right lobe is greater than at the left, depression may be contributing to the client's complaints. Research is continuing to clarify the relationship between emotional characteristics and right frontal-lobe brainwave activity.[15]

We observe differences in brainwave intensity between the frontal lobes in cases in which the client, or parent, reports volatile emotions or, conversely, a too-narrow range of emotions (that is, a monotonic emotional quality, or an emotional flatness). The difference is generally indicated by the increased amplitude of slow-frequency brainwaves (theta and low alpha) in the right frontal lobe. Many other conditions are associated with frontal-lobe imbalances. Experienced neurotherapists can usually describe a client's behavior from the patterns of these imbalances. Some of the major indicators identify confrontational behavior, fibromyalgia and chronic fatigue, emotional volatility, depression, learning disorders, attention difficulties, problems with planning and organizing activities, and problems with motivation and completing tasks.

In the frontal lobes, ideally the amplitude of theta should be about 50 percent greater than the amplitude of beta, with alpha being about 30 percent less than theta. Whatever the ratios for each individual lobe, the lobes should be balanced—that is, the amplitude of each brainwave band should be about the same in each frontal lobe. The rule of thumb for most neurotherapists is that the difference should be less than 10 percent. In my experience, if the difference is greater than about 15 percent, clients admit to the symptoms I have indicated. Detailed descriptions and relevant case examples of many conditions associated with frontal-lobe dysfunction are presented in Chapters 5 and 6.

I have found a similar pattern when the peripheral blood flow between the right and left side of the body is unequal. Peripheral blood flow is a measure of the amount of blood flowing close to the surface of the skin. (I discuss this physiological measure and other forms of biofeedback in Chapter 4.) Peripheral blood flow reflects frontal-cortex activity and is easily measured as hand temperature. While at McLean Hospital, near Boston, and at Harvard Medical School, I collected data on depressed clients at various stages of their hospitalization and treatment. Their depressed states were often worse when the hand temperatures on the right and left were unequal (a difference greater than

3°C.), but they had considerably improved states of mind when their hand temperatures were equal.

Another significant measure taken at the frontal brain sites is the theta/alpha ratio. A high alpha amplitude is associated with a particular form of attention deficiency. The theta/alpha ratio should average about 1.3; a ratio less than 1.0 signals a form of ADD that is usually associated with talkativeness, verbally interruptive behavior, and intellectual flightiness. Individuals with this form of ADD are incessant talkers who constantly interrupt others. They have difficulty following a conversation because they are always anticipating what they will say next. They also tend to have difficulty staying on a specific topic or providing an in-depth analysis of a subject. In school, they catch a snippet of what the teacher says, and then their minds scurry after dozens of associations. They are scattered, disorganized, often dissatisfied with themselves, and frequently depressed.

ADD is believed to be primarily a male disorder, and, indeed, up to four times more males than females are diagnosed with the condition. One unfortunate consequence of this belief is that females with attention deficiencies are often missed. These girls may proceed through their early years doing poorly in school and feeling that they are stupid. I have treated many adult females who were never able to pursue their dreams because of poor academic performance. These women often have the high frontal-lobe alpha pattern of attention deficiency. Because of cultural bias, the behaviors associated with this brain condition (namely, talkativeness and flightiness) are considered feminine. Further, because hyperactivity is not pronounced in this condition, the sufferer is seen by teachers as a nice, polite little girl who is simply not very bright. Because male children are more likely to act out as a result of their attention deficiencies, because of both hormones and cultural expectations, boys are more likely to be seen as problematical and therefore receive attention for their difficulties.

Finally, the measure of summated amplitude ($\Sigma$A) is an important indicator of brain inefficiencies in the frontal areas as well. The sum of the average amplitude of the theta, alpha, and beta bands at these locations should be in the range of 30–60 microvolts. $\Sigma$A much above the 60-microvolt level is often found in cognitively challenged clients, including those with developmental disorders, those with autistic spectrum disorders, and those who are intellectually challenged. When $\Sigma A$ is high over the sensory motor cortex, usually it is high over the frontal lobes as well. Again, high $\Sigma A$ means the various brain locations are not functioning efficiently together.

The wave bands that are measured at the frontal midline (labeled Fz in Figure 2 in Chapter 2) are different from the bands measured at the other locations. Here we measure HF waves at 28–40 Hz, delta waves at 2 Hz, and beta waves at 16–25 Hz. All measurements at this location (as well as at the frontal lobes) are taken with the client's eyes closed. The eyes-closed condition is used to minimize the spikes a neurotherapist often sees in EEG records resulting from eye movement. However, with some children the recordings must be done with eyes open. Autistic children, for example, have great difficulty keeping their eyes closed, and they create more spikes (muscle-movement artifacts) in eyes-closed than in eyes-open states.

The ratio of particular importance at the frontal midline is the HF/beta ratio. The normal range has been found to be between 0.45 and 0.55. Values much above this range indicate obsessive, compulsive, inflexible, and highly repetitive behaviors. Values below this range are associated with excessively passive and indifferent behaviors. The HF/beta ratio, as well as the summated value described in the next paragraph, appears to reflect the activity of the anterior cingulate gyrus. This subcortical structure, discussed earlier, is associated with emotional functions and is implicated in OCD.

Adding the average amplitude of the HF and beta waves is another useful measure because values above 16 microvolts indicate that the person worries and frets. This behavioral pattern appears to be independent of the behaviors associated with the HF/beta ratio. Some people may have obsessive thought patterns but do not admit to excessive worrying. Others who admit to fretting do not consider themselves particularly compulsive or obsessive.

A measurement of delta waves at 2 Hz at the frontal midline appears to be related to chronic pain, intellectual challenge, and an uncommon form of attention deficiency. The quantification of this measure is still under investigation, but at this point amplitudes above 10 microvolts seem to be a cause for concern.

The final measure taken at site Fz is the ratio of slow to fast alpha. The range of slow alpha waves is 8 to 9 Hz, and the range of fast alpha is

11 to 12 Hz. Previously in this chapter I discussed peak alpha frequency, average alpha frequency, and the ratio of slow to fast alpha as important indicators of intellectual performance. Excessive slow-frequency alpha is associated with many problematical conditions, including dementia, schizophrenia, anxiety disorders, and brain injury. Better intellectual performance is directly associated with faster alpha frequencies. For diagnostic purposes, the therapist assesses the simple ratio of the amplitude of the lower frequency to the higher frequency alpha. A ratio above 1.5 is potentially problematical. Values below 1.0 always indicate better intellectual efficiency than do values over 1.5.

What do these measurements mean in practical terms? Ken was a large seventeen-year-old boy who had arrived in my office with the diagnosis of "high functioning autism." He appeared sullen and noncommunicative but quite willing to let me do a brain assessment. I reviewed the results of the assessment with Ken and his mother, and as I usually do, I looked for a positive feature to begin the discussion. In Ken's case I found a low ratio of slow to fast alpha. The ratio was only 0.74, and I told Ken and his mother that this superb ratio was one of the important factors contributing to a high IQ. I also commented on some other positive factors related to this indicator of good cognitive efficiency. Ken was a different boy from that moment on. His mother seemed to be in a state of disbelief, but she managed a weak smile.

Ken flew through his treatments, which consisted entirely of brainwave biofeedback; the HF amplitude was reduced over the frontal midline, and the frontal lobes were normalized. Ken's attention and interpersonal skills improved markedly. His grades became excellent, and he prepared himself to apply to university. Ken started to develop a sense of humor, which is always a strong indicator of improvement in children with autism. He frequently commented to me that he always "felt smart," but people "treated me dumb." This case is an excellent example of the power of revealing positive attributes when a child expects more of the same old criticism of his behavior.

The areas of the brain described in this chapter are the critical "hot spots." Analyzing brainwave activity in these areas helps neurotherapists understand the causes of many disorders. However, the brain is unimaginably complex, and disturbances may reside in many other areas. Further, there can be problems in the way different areas of the brain interact. Neurotherapists can provide complex multisite assessments for determining whether such intersite problems are present. Clinically, however, these five regions reveal most disorders. By carefully assessing these critical areas, neurotherapists can, with remarkable accuracy, specify the symptoms for which the client is seeking treatment. The other important advantage of the assessment of these critical areas is that an experienced neurotherapist can accomplish the assessment and do a thorough review of the brainwave results with a client in a single one-hour session. With the assessment completed, a neurotherapist can show the client where in the brain the cause of the problems resides and can explain the specific treatment that will improve the client's condition. If you recognize your own, a family member's, or a client's ailments in the descriptions in this chapter, neurotherapy may be able to help. Along the way to a cure neurotherapists have many tools at their disposal, as described in the next chapter.

CHAPTER 4

# Neurotherapy and Its Partners in Treatment

As the field of neurotherapy has grown, so have the tools that allow neurotherapists to help people. Of the many different forms of neurotherapy, neurofeedback is the most promising for a number of conditions. In my experience, neurofeedback is the most important ingredient in the mix, though other interventions can be added to improve outcomes or to speed the process. In neurofeedback, you can receive instant information about brain activity from a specific brain area, though the activity cannot be directly felt. You can then use that information to learn how to self-regulate your brain's activity.

To know where in the brain neurofeedback would be useful, neurotherapists produce a brain map, based on an EEG recording. They compare the EEG data with normative data bases that precisely identify those regions in the brain that are not functioning within normal limits. The power of neurotherapy to treat a wide range of disorders results directly from the brain map–based diagnosis. The brain map specifies what the problem is and where in the brain the problem resides. Treatment goals, therefore, are straightforward. Yet straightforward does not necessarily imply easy or rapid. Some brain activity and some regions of the brain are less amenable to change and more difficult to train than others. That is why additional forms of neurotherapy have been developed as supplements to neurofeedback, which is the backbone of neurotherapeutic treatment. The added treatments are likewise targeted at specific brain areas or brain functions. And neurotherapists know that the treatments are effective for a specific client because they pretest them when the client's EEG is being monitored. In short, therapists know precisely what a treatment will do because they see the effects on the brain monitor.

Many complementary treatments are used in neurotherapy. All stimulation influences the brain. Sounds, for example, affect the brain in ways we can monitor on the EEG. Similarly, light, electrical stimulation, vibration, and visual images with different content, such as pleasing or repulsive photographs, all can spark activity in specific brain areas. Audiovisual devices that stimulate with light and sound in specific wave lengths are particularly effective for children with reading problems and the elderly who are starting to show mental sluggishness. Cranial microamperage stimulators, electrical devices that stimulate the brain, are useful for anxious, depressed, and sleep-disturbed clients. Harmonic sounds below the threshold of hearing enhance or suppress the brainwaves that are being modified. In neurotherapy, biofeedback is not limited to the brain. Biofeedback of heart rate, skin conductance, muscle tension, skin temperature, and respiration are adjuncts to neurotherapy that help regularize the functioning of the nervous system.

The course of treatment for disorders may, therefore, include procedures other than neurofeedback. I cover five types of these procedures in this chapter. First, as many of the cases in this book show, sometimes psychotherapy is needed to help clients sort through the psychological baggage and family dynamics that accompany many disorders. Certain clients, such as victims of traumatic stress, may need quite a lot of psychotherapy or family therapy, whereas others require little or none. Second, certain procedures are designed to nudge, or stimulate, the brain. Third, many neurotherapists also include other supportive treatments. Peripheral biofeedback, for example, can be an important additional therapy. Some neurotherapists are also practitioners of subtle therapeutic energy techniques. These include a wide range of procedures including hypnosis, Qi gong, healing or therapeutic touch, audiovisual stimulation, meridian-based techniques including acupuncture and acustimulation, craniosacral therapy, and a variety of energy-psychology techniques. The additional procedures that I use in my clinic include neuroactive harmonic sounds, energy-psychology techniques, audiovisual stimulation, acustimulation, and craniosacral therapy. Fourth, two other levels of neurotherapy—preventative maintenance and peak-performance training—are designed to maintain and enhance gains clients make with neurofeedback. Fifth, home treatments are used as adjuncts to accelerate neurotherapy and to sustain the gains made during treatment.

We turn our attention now to the mix of the various therapies that are combined in treating many disorders. Let's start with the most important treatment of all.

## Neurofeedback

Neurofeedback, also called brainwave feedback or brainwave biofeedback, is the fundamental treatment method in neurotherapy. In principal, neurofeedback is simple. When the brain is doing what is desired, the client hears a tone or sees an object move on a computer monitor (or both). She makes use of this information to learn how to modify brainwave activity, which occurs at a level that is too subtle for her to feel. This subtleness makes biofeedback a powerful treatment procedure. We can monitor, and learn to control, changes in neurological activity at levels well below those a person can sense.

When working with adults, neurotherapists tend to use sounds and moving graph presentations on a computer monitor as the training feedback signals. For example, to teach you how to increase theta amplitude, a neurotherapist configures the software so that you can see the theta-band activity on the computer monitor. When the amplitude goes above a set training threshold, a sound comes on. You are then instructed to "try to keep the tone on." Often clients ask, "How do I keep the tone on?" Basically, it is an intuitive process in which the normal mentally driven fluctuation in brainwave amplitude is reinforced by the feedback tone. The client comes to identify the subjective mental state that coincides with the feedback and hence is able to prolong the time in that state as guided by the feedback. This process is to some extent unconscious, so clients in fuguelike and comalike states can be treated with tones as well. The tone coinciding with the desired state increases the time in that state even for clients in these mentally compromised conditions.

Each treatment session usually lasts forty minutes and is broken into four to eight individual trials, or epochs. You "work" for five minutes to try to keep the tone on. At the end of the five-minute trial, the average theta amplitude is recorded, and the next trial starts. The training threshold is set so that the tone remains on about 70 percent of the time—that is, the theta amplitude is maintained above the set threshold 70 percent of the time. As training proceeds and the amplitude stays above the threshold more than 70 percent of the time, say 90 percent, the neurotherapist increases the training threshold to maximize the learning opportunities. Thus, you learn to keep the theta amplitude at higher and higher levels as training proceeds. Once you learn how to control brainwave amplitude at one level, the therapist increases the difficulty of the training. In small increments, your brainwave amplitudes change in the desired direction.

When working with children, neurotherapists use simplified feedback. The software is set up so that the children are essentially playing a video game with their brains. Neurotherapists use many different types of displays, but basically when the amplitude of the brainwave under training moves in the desired direction, a figure moves on the computer monitor. The Pac-Man display used with one particular brand of software is a good example. When the theta amplitude, for example, falls below the training threshold, Pac-Man chews up dots on the screen. Pac-Man's progress in chewing up dots starts and stops depending on the brainwave amplitude. Many different game displays have been developed for neurotherapy. The child can fly aircraft, make Superman or Superwoman fly, make a clownlike figure move up or down, move balloons around the screen, and so on. The video game should not be too exciting. If the purpose of the brainwave training is to increase focus and attention, the game itself must not interfere with that training by being inherently exciting enough to sustain the child's focus. In such a situation the child is not learning to focus her attention. We do make the game somewhat interesting by providing the child with a score, just as in regular video games. In the balloon game, for example, the score increases every time the child moves a balloon around a specific path on the screen.

Inexperienced neurotherapists can make a serious mistake when treating children with ADD by providing too much variety and stimulation. Easily bored, the child may play one game for a brief period of time, announce that he is bored and ask the therapist for a new game. Then, quickly bored with the second game, the child asks for yet another one, and so on. In this situation, the neurotherapist has inadvertently become part of the problem for which the child is being treated. Changing the stimulus in an effort to sustain the child's focus is inefficient and often results in the failure of the therapy, which is intended to enhance the child's capacity for stable attention. Experienced therapists give the child a limited choice of activities and then gently, but emphatically, restrict the child's activity to the chosen alternative.

The child's attention is sustained and reinforced by coaching, shaping, and regulating the length of each training epoch. The child may start with epochs only three to five minutes in length. The therapist engages the child in keeping score and, when possible, noting and recording the brainwave data. As the session progresses, the therapist verbally rewards the child for her progress and announces when it is appropriate to increase the difficulty of the game. The relationship of brain activity to the game activity and score is explained at an age-appropriate level, and the child is also involved in setting the epoch length. "You did very well for three minutes. How long should we make the game this time?" By engaging the child in these activities the therapist shapes the child's attention and strongly facilitates the training of brain activity.

It is critical that the child and, particularly, the parent not be focused exclusively on the brainwave data from session to session. Parents often want to see the child's brain activity improve markedly each time. When they do not see improvement, they may discourage the child ("You did not do well today, you must try harder"). This is precisely the same discouraging situation that the child likely already faces in school or at home because of his ADD condition. In the neurotherapy session, the child can always have a successful experience because the therapist can adjust the brainwave threshold required for the reward. By analogy, if a high jumper is clearing the bar only 40 percent of the time on a particular day, the bar can be lowered so that the jumper clears the bar 80 percent of the time. The object is to maximize the positive learning opportunities within each session.

To parents, I explain that progress in neurotherapy can look like changes in the stock market during prosperous times. The general trend of the market is up, but there are major day-to-day fluctuations. I also show the parents data of successfully treated clients whose session-to-session scores show these variations. Sometimes parents are quite resistant to the notion that their child can be making significant progress even though the brainwave scores are not changing or perhaps are even becoming worse over the course of a few sessions.

One day Niki, a seven-year-old girl with ADD and below-grade-level reading, seemed withdrawn, quite different from her usual bouncy self. The neurotherapist on this occasion was our reading specialist, who had good rapport with this child, and she was struck by Niki's change in attitude. On previous visits, Niki seemed to be happy; she was cooperative and highly interactive with the neurotherapist. But on this occasion she sat sad-faced and quite still. The neurotherapist made gentle inquiries, but Niki responded with shrugs of her shoulders or clipped answers of "yes" or "no" or "I don't know." The mystery was solved when the mother entered the treatment room toward the end of the session and curtly said to Niki, "I hope you did better. It is a long drive down here."

Sometimes neurotherapists have to be blunt with parents whose behavior is interfering with the child's progress. In this case I asked to see the mother alone and showed her the data from several cases of successful treatments where the initial neurological data were negative. I said I needed her commitment to give the treatment a chance. It was critical that she remain positive, complimentary, and supportive of Niki's efforts during the sessions. She had to praise Niki for a job well done after every session, regardless of her own feelings about how well Niki had performed. I further asked her to agree that she would not see any of Niki's data for the next few sessions. Niki's mother was a bright, caring, and intuitive woman who instantly grasped the problem. She agreed with my recommendations, and the case turned out very well indeed. After five more sessions, Niki asked whether she could take home the book she had been reading during the neurotherapy/remediation session because she wanted to finish the story. This request was a huge breakthrough for this previously poor reader, and her mother tearfully related her shock when Niki read parts of the book on the long drive home. At that same session, Niki asked to show her mother the brainwave data, which had shown a major positive shift in amplitude.

Children seem to be much less fixated than their parents on the neurological data even though they help the neurotherapist calculate the numbers several times during each session. When a child does seem inordinately interested, the therapist usually has a frank discussion with the parent about taking precautions to prevent the child from becoming discouraged with the treatment. When talking to a child, I often use an analogy of a game such as baseball. A baseball team may have scored five runs in one game, two in the next, ten in the third, and just one run in the fourth game. However, the team may have won all four games because they played better than the opposing team. In the neurotherapy sessions, the child is encouraged to focus on the score, recognizing that the score is going to vary as we make the sessions longer or shorter and as we make the game harder by requiring ever greater periods of concentration to get the screen icon to move. Most children understand that a score of fifty points in an easy game is easier to get than a score of ten in a hard game.

The conditions required for positive feedback in a neurotherapy session can be made straightforward, as in the above examples, or complex. For example, the feedback can be regulated so that the sounds occur or the screen icons move whenever theta amplitude falls below the set threshold. The feedback condition can be set so that two or three different brainwave-band amplitudes must be above their individual thresholds for feedback to occur. One brainwave-band amplitude might have to be below a threshold and a second brainwave-band amplitude above a different threshold for feedback to occur. Ratios are also used, which might, for example, require one wave-band amplitude to be a certain amount greater than a second wave-band amplitude. Different areas of the brain can be monitored simultaneously. Four different feedback tones can each indicate a brainwave activity at a different location.

The relationships among different parts of the brain can also be the focus of neurofeedback training. Neurotherapists refer to such intersite relationships as "the brain talking to itself." The brainwave feedback can be activated by the relationship of brainwave amplitudes at two different sites. Coherence refers to the degree to which brainwave amplitudes and frequencies in different parts of the brain move in unison—that is, the waves are in phase. Complete (100 percent) coherence occurs when the phases of a particular brainwave band at two sites are perfectly correlated. The two sites in such a situation are completely interdependent. However, high levels of intersite coherence are generally not a desired brain state. When working with difficult problems such as traumatic brain injury, seizure disorders, or psychoses, the specific nature of the two-site relationship can be quite complex. Feedback can be set to occur, for example, only when the phase of a specific frequency is moving in unison at two sites. Further, the parameters can be set so that the shape and phase of a brainwave at two different sites must have a specific shared pattern for a tone to occur. Suffice it to say, the methods of biofeedback now form an array of possibilities to meet the different needs of diverse clients.

## Treating Psychological and Social Problems

The major barriers to success faced by the neurotherapist are not those of correcting or optimizing brain functioning. Although some brain activities are more difficult to modify than others, generally the brain responds to treatment remarkably well. The principal problems neurotherapists face are psychological and social.

### Psychotherapy

Everyone has problems, or psychological baggage, and resolving these issues is the focus of psychotherapy. In the context of neurotherapy, all brainwave anomalies are accompanied by psychological consequences. If neurotherapeutic treatment is unsuccessful, usually the neurotherapist has not effectively addressed the client's psychological issues and complicating social relationships. In general, psychological baggage consists of mental and physical habits that are established to defend the psychological identity and integrity of the person, his family, or his significant peer group. If John feels stupid because his attention wanders, any number of possible psychological defences may become established. He may simply give up and refuse to do schoolwork because, psychologically, it is less damaging to be regarded as obstinate than as stupid.

The major problem with these habitual patterns is that they can become ingrained. Thus, after the fundamental cause of the problem is resolved, the pattern may continue because of independent social reinforcement. For example, John may receive considerable attention for his defiant behavior. This attention strongly reinforces the behavior. Further, if the pattern is developed to avoid or minimize severe negative emotions, such as fear or humiliation, then the pattern can become deep-seated because the negative emotion and its associated thought system are never tested for validity relative to current reality. So even if

John's neurological problem is corrected, he may continue to refuse to do well in school because of previously experienced fear or humiliation.

**FREQUENTLY ASKED QUESTION**

Q: My nine-year-old son has been kicked out of school again for fighting and disrupting the class. How can neurotherapy make a difference?

A: Neurotherapy alone probably will not be adequate because the defensive aggressive behavior must be modified. Neurotherapy can correct the neurological bases of the problem, and then family or behavior therapy can modify your son's destructive behavior.

As I like to say to neurotherapist trainees, a client sent from heaven is a seven-year-old girl with ADD without hyperactivity (now called ADHD, Inattentive Type) whose family is intact and genuinely supportive of the child. Their love of their daughter is unconditional, and she knows that being loved by her parents is not dependent on her achievements. I can virtually guarantee that this child will be successfully treated and achieving at grade level within fifteen to twenty sessions. A client from hell is a forty-year-old male with unresolved ADD who has been routinely unsuccessful at keeping a job or sustaining a meaningful relationship. He is depressed, alcoholic or drug-addicted, and on some form of public assistance. He has had numerous experiences with various therapies, all unsuccessful. A less extreme version is the marginally successful male who has problems with his relationships and presents himself as just a "laid-back, disorganized, easy-going, motivationally limited kind of guy." These clients have acquired enormous psychological baggage, which proves far more problematic to deal with than any neurological inefficiencies.

Clients with significant psychological baggage are usually pessimistic and often are committed to their disabled personal states. At the simplest level, those on disability-based financial support often find the prospect of functioning independently overwhelming. They have to make considerable effort and marked changes in lifestyle to achieve the same economic well-being as an independently functioning person. These clients are vigilant for signs of therapeutic failure. When requested to do routine monitoring of their symptoms or activities, they usually do not comply and offer only global reports of "no noticeable changes." They engage therapists in irrelevant discussions or attempt to turn the discussion to elaborate tales of their psychological woes. Such clients look for therapeutic contradictions by asking the same question at different times or of different therapists, and then they point out the apparent inconsistencies in the responses to their queries. All these behaviors are defensive and serve to protect the client from feared changes to the status quo. Therapists who are unsuccessful are often tempted to blame the client. After all, they clearly are committed to their present condition, get reinforcement from the situation, and appear to simply not want to "get better."

A message on my answering machine sounded tearfully joyous. "Dr. Swingle, I just want to thank you so much. After my first treatment yesterday, I experienced something I never experienced before in my life—a complete absence of fear. I was able to leave the [place where she was staying] and walk down the hill all by myself, and I wasn't afraid. Thank you so much, and I look forward to our next session and starting a new life." I congratulated myself for choosing an aggressive first neurotherapeutic treatment for Jill, a severely dysfunctional woman. Yet she never came for further treatments. She returned to her hospital day-care program, and when I called her, she said that she couldn't "arrange" for treatments, even though the treatment facility was on hospital grounds. Jill's psychiatrist later said that, in her opinion, Jill simply could not handle the changes that recovery would entail. I often play the recording of Jill's message on my answering machine at training workshops that I present for neurotherapists. Jill's case represents a failure of judgment on my part because I did not heed the warning signs of a client with severe psychological baggage acquired from years of chronic anxiety. I have heard that Sigmund Freud once told a trainee, "Don't cure the headache until you cure the problem." Clients whose chronic conditions have remained essentially unchanged for many years wrap their entire lives around the disorder. The disorder is the focus of their conversations. They become "experts" in the disorder and "experts" in treatments that are largely ineffective. The secondary gains of a chronic disorder often include avoidance of responsibilities and control over others. Such clients present major challenges that go far beyond the realm of neurotherapy.

A related form of excessive baggage often occurs in the chronically disabled client who also suffers from a personality disorder. The combination pattern can arise in several ways. For example, an adult woman may have developed fibromyalgia after a series of traumas. Fibromyalgia is characterized by chronic pain that usually moves about the body. The pain, in turn, results in sleep disturbances, which lead to other problems such as chronic fatigue, mood swings, and intensified pain. Fibromyalgia is also often associated with attention, focus, and comprehension problems. "Fibrofog" limits the client's ability to sustain employment or other artistic or intellectual pursuits. The fibromyalgia client is generally depressed and often ingests huge quantities of medications. Fibromyalgia is usually found in people with a history of physical or psychological trauma. A physical injury sustained in an automobile accident is a common precipitating event. Other common causes include psychological trauma (for example, an abusive relationship), severe viral infection, or autoimmune forms of arthritis. If the client has developed a personality disorder as a result of early psychological trauma, the combination of chronic pain and a personality disorder can render the client severely resistant to treatment.

Personality disorders incorporate negative core beliefs about the self. The emotion-laden beliefs can include feelings that one is worthless, unlovable, evil, stupid, loathsome, and disgusting. These debilitating feelings can result in behaviors that are barriers to successful therapy. These clients need ever-expanding evidence that they are special (such as demanding additional therapeutic time, phoning about "emergencies," or expressing desperate needs for information). Their need to feel loved may take the form of persistent probing as to the therapist's feelings about them. Personality-disordered clients often perceive therapy as a source of love, security, and friendship rather than as a way to solve their problems. These clients "collect" therapists; they sustain a love/hate relationship with therapists whom they often maintain are extremely helpful and talented despite the fact that their condition remains largely unchanged.

Sometimes it is best if this sort of client works with two therapists, one focusing on changing the brainwave activity and the second working with the emotional issues, some of which can be at least temporarily worsened in the course of the neurotherapy. As an example, a client with early-childhood issues is likely to find that emotions related to those early problem rise to the surface of consciousness in the course of slow-wave enhancement. One possible reason is that children have greater theta brainwave states than adults, and the early-childhood experiences are associated with theta activity. When theta amplitude is enhanced in neurotherapy, the emotional power of these previous memories is intensified. Helping the client work through these wrenching memories may be done by the neurotherapist if properly trained or by a psychotherapist, although clients often resolve many of these emotional issues alone without any professional assistance. The pacing of the neurotherapy sessions can itself be important in that clients need adequate time to deal with the emotional content of the resurrected memories.

By all appearances, Luke seemed to be happy, jovial, and socially outgoing. He dressed in a sort of crumpled manner and identified himself as an artist who had "lost it—or maybe never had it." Luke loved to be in therapy. If possible, he would have come seven days a week. He thought I did "great work." Unfortunately, he did not improve in any meaningful way. He still spent most of the day in bed and most of the night in front of the TV. His apartment, he said, was "absolutely filthy" with "months" of dirty dishes and take-out containers piled everywhere. He kept a studio in his apartment that he had avoided for "years." Of Luke's many neurological inefficiencies, one marked problem was a severe deficiency of theta amplitude in the back of the brain. After a number of training sessions, Luke's theta amplitude began to increase. On one occasion, when the theta amplitude had increased considerably, Luke started to hyperventilate, and it looked as though he was about to have a full-blown panic attack. When he recovered, he started to tell me of a period during his childhood in which he was ritually abused by his father. He never had forgotten his father beating him and locking him in a closet, but the memories seemed not to be real. It was "sort of like watching a movie in a detached state of mind." This session marked the turning point in Luke's treatment. We dealt with the abuse among many other issues during ongoing neurotherapy to normalize the brain. Luke is back to painting, but he maintains that he will never be able to support himself with his artwork alone. At present he works as a security guard.

To return to the treatment of children, most of these cases are not as serious as adult cases. We have youth on our side when we treat children. Their brains are more susceptible to change than are adult brains, and, more important, whatever excess baggage they have acquired lacks the chronic element and reinforced behaviors and habits that develop over time. Their excess baggage most frequently comes in three forms: low self-esteem, destructive behavior, and family dynamics (which are discussed in the next section).

I often say to parents, "If you fix self-esteem, you fix a lot of problems." Nothing is as sad as seeing a young child who is embarrassed to be who she is. These children are withdrawn and feel worthless. Despite supportive efforts of parents, they are often ridiculed because of learning problems. Clearly the longer this pattern continues, the more severe the erosion of their self-esteem. One of the most thrilling experiences of a neurotherapist is to witness the transformation that takes place when a demoralized child gains a significant belief in his or her self-worth.

An important aspect of neurotherapy with these children is providing them with experiences of success. These experiences can take many forms, and some require only the authoritative statement of "the doctor." For example, when I measure the brain map of a child, I often find a feature that can provide an anchor for positive self-esteem. Sheila had the form of ADD that manifests itself only during a cognitive challenge (such as reading) and only over the sensory motor cortex, at the top of the brain. The brain activity across all other brain locations looked fine, including low theta/beta ratios in the frontal areas. I told Sheila that her brain got mixed up and was sending out daydreaming messages when she wanted to read. All we had to do was help her teach her brain to send out the correct brainwaves when she wanted to read. I also told her that the front of her brain was producing the activity of a "rocket scientist." The mother later told me that the transformation in her child's orientation toward schoolwork was simply remarkable after she reported to her family that she had the brain of a rocket scientist. This child successfully completed treatment in thirteen sessions.

Another brainwave signature that creates positive self-esteem is the artist's signature, which, as shown in Chapter 1 with Jason, is high alpha-wave increases at the back and on the top of the brain immediately after the child's eyes are closed. When I see this pattern, I ask the children whether they like art or building things, and I almost always get an affirmative response. I then proceed to explain the significance of the artist's signature and refer to the children as young Picassos or another artist whose name they recognize.

Positive brainwave patterns are not found routinely, so the neurotherapist must find other ways for the child to be positively acknowledged and to experience success. Examples include praising her for taking less time to do her homework, reporting positive comments from teachers, or expressing approval when she reads or does other scholastic activities on her own. If the neurotherapist is vigilant about praising such progress, the child's self-esteem can be boosted while the brainwave treatment is proceeding.

Excess baggage that takes the form of defiant, disruptive, or destructive behavior can be complicated to treat. Oppositional defiance disorder (ODD) is a complex problem in that, in addition to the behavioral components, it is often associated with inefficiencies in the frontal lobes of the brain. Nina Lindberg and her colleagues at the University of Helsinki in Finland studied the relationship between brain dysfunction and aggression.[1] They reported that homicidal men, schizophrenics, and children diagnosed with ODD and conduct disorder had considerably more indicators of brain dysfunction than did control subjects. These negative behavior patterns are acquired and then carried on; they are not caused by specific brain inefficiency, dysfunction, or damage. In many cases, boys adopt hostile attitudes in order to defend against feelings of profound inadequacy. These feelings, in turn, can have many causes. To take the most straightforward example, a male child with a learning disorder such as ADHD may find relief from his feelings of being stupid, coupled with the profound discomfort caused by lack of stimulation, by being vigorously disruptive in school, at home, and in social situations such as group play. Strongly reinforced by the stimulating effects of his disruptive behavior and the attention such behavior gains him, the pattern becomes ingrained and persists even after brainwave modification is successful. Often these children refuse to participate in neurotherapeutic sessions. Behavioral therapy is always required with these children in conjunction with the neurotherapy. It is a positive indicator when the disruptive child cooperates with the neurotherapist, whatever apparent indifference the child may exhibit.

### Family Therapy

Family therapists maintain that all disorders are family disorders, including alcoholism, depression, cancer, and certainly a child's learning problems. The need for therapies supportive of the neurotherapeutic changes in these cases has been emphasized by many professionals. At some point during neurotherapy and behavior therapy, it is helpful for the family as a whole to receive treatment.

In the 1998 National Institutes of Health *Consensus Statement* on the diagnosis and treatment of ADHD, the authors point out that the ADHD child's hyperactivity, academic underachievement, and related problems of drug abuse, antisocial behavior, defiance, and increased proneness to all sorts of injuries severely affect family life.[2] Compared with parents who do not have children with ADHD, parents of an ADHD child experience greater marital discord and higher divorce rates as a result of family stress. This family strife further exacerbates the ADHD of the child because of increased stress levels. In addition, the disruptive behavior of the child often stirs strong animosity and resentment in the family. The friction can be blatant or quite subtle. I have had cases in which parents bluntly announce that they are considering putting their child up for adoption or placing their child in foster care. This announcement has on occasion been made in the presence of the child! Such complicated and dysfunctional family dynamics should be mediated by a skilled family therapist. If needed, the family therapist should be independent of the neurotherapy clinic, and that person should be viewed as unaligned with any family member. I also am encouraged when the child agrees with the suggestion that family counseling will help resolve the family's problems.

Problems with family dynamics are not necessarily initially obvious in these situations. Most emerge subtly as neurotherapy proceeds. Two forms are quite common. First, a resentful parent may allow the neurotherapy to continue but nonetheless hold to the conviction that the child's problems in school simply reflect laziness, purposeful defiance, or ungratefulness (it is the child's "fault"). The consistent message the child receives is that even though his condition is improving, these changes could have been accomplished anyway (with a lot less hassle and expense) if he had not been so lazy. This destructive dynamic is most often found between a father and a son. Although family therapy would be useful in such cases, I often find that the parent refuses to participate. Neurotherapy can be successful even in these circumstances, but the child's future accomplishments are always tainted by the parent's unresolved and inappropriate resentment.

The second family dynamic that can limit the success of neurotherapy arises when the child's disorder is of central importance to the integrity of the family structure. This dynamic can take several forms. In split or blended families the child's disorder intensifies in response to the restructuring of the family unit. On the surface it seems that the child is attempting to disrupt the new relationship, either by requiring increasing amounts of attention (as in the inability to do homework independently) or by requiring increasing discipline for disruptive behavior. Such changes in the family structure are always frightening, painful, and confusing to the child and frequently result in feelings of guilt or abandonment or both. The child's school problems can have secondary reinforcing properties because they increase adult attention and thereby reduce the feelings of abandonment and powerlessness.

Another common form of family dysfunction arises when one family member is caring for a disabled partner. The relationship gains meaning from the care giving and would be forced to go through feared and uncomfortable changes, or even disintegrate, if the disabled person became capable of functioning independently. Likewise, when a marriage is in jeopardy, the disability of a child can provide the narrow focus of common concern required to distract the couple from their marital discord. If the child improves and becomes capable of being independent, the parents are confronted with the loss of purpose and meaning necessary for maintaining their relationship.

Other variations of family dysfunction exist. How conscious family members are of the dysfunctional dynamics varies. In some cases, none of the family members appear to be aware of the pattern that has been established. In this situation the child cannot improve because such a change would result in the destruction of the family unit. Another frequent variation is the parents' refusing to acknowledge positive changes in a child. I have had cases in which the child reports improvements, which are validated by teachers' comments and markedly improved grades, but the parent persists in wanting to pursue alternative and often aggressive treatment for a learning problem that no longer exists. In one case, following a report card that contained only As and Bs, the mother asked, "Isn't there anything we can do about Joe's attention deficit disorder?" This was one of the few occasions on which I administered an attention-assessment test. I had the child take the computerized Connor's

Continuous Performance Test. The test showed that he had no attention deficiencies.

Another variation occurs when ADHD evolves into defiance and conduct disorders, a common outcome. Although prescription drugs may help temporarily by improving attention and dampening the disruptive/inattentive behavior, medication does not get at the root causes of attentional and behavioral problems. A pill does not teach a child how to interact with others. An early review by James Satterfield reported on studies showing that individuals with ADHD and ODD placed on Ritalin alone (that is, with no supportive therapies) had poor long-term outcomes.[3] He further reported that many incarcerated offenders with a history of ADHD had been placed on medication only, without supportive therapies. Joel Lubar of the University of Tennessee and Judith Lubar of the Southeastern Biofeedback and Neurobehavioral Institute in Knoxville likewise caution that with neurotherapy long-term behavioral changes are unlikely to persist unless the neurotherapy is integrated with other remedial programs and therapies, such as family therapy.[4]

Therapy for family problems takes many different forms. Sometimes the therapist works only with the parents, sometimes with a parent and one child, and sometimes with everyone. For a problem of resentment, a therapist generally sees the resentful parent alone and then the parent with the child. Sometimes the problems can be worked out quickly. For example, Charles, the father of Sam, resented the fact that he had to pay for Sam's neurotherapy treatments for ADD. Charles maintained that if Sam only "applied himself," he would not need the treatments. Chapter 5 of this book contains the partial text of a recorded interview with Roy, a father with ADD. Roy described the terrible pain he felt as a child with ADD. He wanted to spare his son the pain he had endured as a child. I have Roy's permission to use his recorded account for clinical purposes, and I played the tape for Charles. After Charles recovered from his sobbing, I reviewed with him the positive and supportive things he could do to help his son. The most critical one was for Charles to praise and hug Sam for every imaginable reason, and if he could not think of a reason, to hug him anyway. I then met with Charles and Sam together and worked out Sam's homework schedule. Sam agreed to ask his father for help with homework when he got stuck. Sam received extra help at school and had a tutor to help with his homework. His mother was also supportive and helped Sam with his homework. Charles's resentment was based on an inadequate understanding of the neurological conditions contributing to Sam's problems, and the resentment was resolved quickly once Charles listened to Roy describe his personal experiences with ADD.

## Nudging the Brain

The problems that people bring to the neurotherapist can be thought of as indicators that the brain is stuck in a particular suboptimal pattern. In this condition, the brain's range of activity is narrow or highly repetitive, for example. The purpose of nudging techniques is to "unstick" the brain and increase the range and flexibility of brain activity. Basically these procedures are computer programs that direct the brain to act certain ways. Less Draconian than they sound, these procedures can be thought of as brain exercisers. At present only a few such systems exist, but this area of neurotherapy is vigorously developing and may eventually evolve into a fundamental form of practice.

### Brain Disentrainment
One system is called brain disentrainment, and several variations have been developed. This procedure first measures the dominant brainwave frequency at a particular location. Based on that measurement, it stimulates the brain at a frequency that is a bit above or below that of the dominant frequency. What is *dominant frequency*? Brainwaves vary in electrical strength (measured in microvolts) across all frequencies. One point on that frequency spectrum, in each measurement sample, is the strongest, and the frequency at that highest voltage point is the dominant frequency. The average of, say, one hundred such measurements, which might require only a few seconds of data recording, reveals the dominant frequency.

Based on that rate, the brain is then given light, sound, electromagnetic, or microamperage (low electrical) stimulation at a frequency slightly greater or less than the dominant frequency. For example, if a therapist wants to stimulate the brain at 10 percent slower than the dominant frequency, and that frequency is 10 Hz, then for one second the stimulation rate will be 9 Hz. This sequence continues with the stimulation frequency changing every second or so for the entire time of treatment to nudge the brain to increase the range of the dominant frequency. Light stimulation is usually delivered by very small lights called light emitting diodes (LEDs) that are fixed to eyeglass frames. With eyes usually closed, these lights directly stimulate the brain. When using lights with delayed-development or autistic children, eyeglass frames usually cannot be used early in treatment because the child cannot tolerate the procedure. In such cases we use strobe-type light fixtures that are not worn by the child but rather are handheld like a flashlight.

One autistic child, Billy, finally learned to tolerate the electrodes on his head and ears after his parents made a game of putting on the electrodes at home while giving Billy treats such as cookies. Billy, however, would have nothing to do with the eyeglass frames with the lights. He would yank them off unless his father held his arms. Billy rapidly learned to shake his head vigorously to remove the glasses, and his distress was such that we abandoned the glasses in favor of the strobe light. This device can be used in various ways. We had Billy sit in his father's lap while his father read a story to him. I held the strobe light so it reflected off the pages of the book while Billy was looking at the pictures. While we were using the strobe, both I and Billy's father wore the glass frames with the flashing lights. Eventually Billy wanted to try the glasses, and we slowly increased the time Billy wore the glasses for treatment.

Sound stimulation is usually supplied via headphones, but, as with the use of a handheld strobe light for autistic children, it can be delivered through external speakers. The frequency of the sound is varied either with repetitive beeps (such as a tone beeping at 10 Hz) or with blended tones that produce a beat frequency. For example, a combination of two tones, one at 300 Hz and the second at 310 Hz produces a beat frequency heard at 10 Hz. If one listens to a 10-Hz beat frequency, the amplitude of the 10-Hz (alpha) brainwave increases. Clients often find that listening to 10-Hz tones has a relaxing effect because of the increased alpha in the brain.

### Brainwave Suppression

Sometimes toward the end of a trying day when I have seen only defiant and uncooperative children, fate gives me a reprieve. One day that reprieve was Lucy, an eight-year-old sweetheart. "Hi, Dr. Swingle" was music to my ears as she hopped into the treatment chair. "Today I'm going to take the blue agate from the treasure box. Is it still there?" "If it's gone, we'll find another one," I replied. "Am I going to hear that funny sound again today?" she asked, and I told her she indeed would be using the headsets again and hearing the sound every once in a while. The sound that Lucy heard was a whooshing sound. Embedded were tones too low in amplitude for her to pick out of the whooshing sound. The particular blend of sounds embedded in the whooshing sound suppressed theta amplitude and helped Lucy stay focused when she started to drift. The sound was low, so it was not irritating, but it increased the efficiency of the neurofeedback session in training the brain. Sound stimulation is used to help a child maintain focus. If we want to talk with the child, have the child read, or need strong stimulation for focus, we tend to use lights. In both cases the goal is to augment the neurofeedback sessions, and the use of these additives is slowly reduced over time.

**FREQUENTLY ASKED QUESTION**

Q: I have severe headaches. Can neurotherapy help?

A: Neurotherapy can be helpful for severe chronic headaches. For less severe conditions, there may be more efficient alternatives, such as relaxation training, muscle (EMG) biofeedback, and hand-temperature biofeedback.

### Electromagnetic and Microamperage Stimulation

The famous psychologist and philosopher William James suggested a diagnostic category that I find truly captures the torment of some clients. He called this condition "torn-to-pieces-hood," by which he meant an acute state of anxiety, despair, and hopelessness. Many clients desperate to find relief fit this category perfectly. They are treated assertively with brain-driving techniques that use electromagnetic and microamperage electrical stimulation. Electromagnetic stimulation is delivered with small stimulators placed on the head. Microamperage stimulation is applied either about the head or on acupuncture points. The stimulation is weak, at a level that is just below the feeling threshold.

Agatha was in acute torn-to-pieces-hood. She felt that everything was crashing in on her. "I just can't cope," she cried. "I can't go on meds and turn into an addicted zombie again and have those other problems."

She had complained of a number of side effects with antianxiety medications, including intestinal problems, fatigue, and mental fogginess. When a client is in severe distress, the neurotherapist has to calm the overall autonomic nervous system as well as the brain. In Chinese medicine, the emergency acupuncture point is located under the nose, so I stimulated that point with a brief electrical pulse. I then put stick-on electrodes over several acupuncture points on the forearms, lower legs, and hands. With sticky tape I attached small electromagnets (about the size of a stack of three dimes) to two locations on Agatha's head. The magnets and electrodes attached were being controlled by the theta amplitude in the back of her brain. When the amplitude dropped, the stimulators were engaged and drove up the amplitude. When the amplitude was up, Agatha heard a pleasant tone, and she was instructed to allow the tone to be on as often as she could manage. I told her to "let it happen; don't try to make it happen." The brain-driving electrical and magnetic stimulation helped Agatha with the neurofeedback by driving up the theta anytime it remained too low for a period of time. Most clients respond rapidly to this assertive treatment, and, fortunately, Agatha found rapid relief from her physiological distress with this approach. We then continued with her neurofeedback treatments to normalize her brainwave patterns, thereby increasing her stress tolerance.

---

**FREQUENTLY ASKED QUESTION**

Q: My daughter is autistic. We saw a brainwave therapist, but my daughter could not pay attention to the feedback displays. How can neurotherapy help a severe case of autism?

A: New technologies have been developed that are nonvolitional, meaning that we stimulate the brain even if the child is not attentive. I start with these brain-driving procedures, and then, as the child's symptoms improve and she can pay attention, I switch to biofeedback.

---

### Braindryvr

Another brain-nudging system increases or decreases the amplitude of specific brainwave bands. The system, developed in my clinic, is called the Braindryvr. This machine makes use of sound stimulation. Sound stimulation that, for example, suppresses the amplitude of theta brainwaves is switched on or off as a direct result of the changes in the client's theta activity. To decrease theta amplitude at the top of the head, the system is calibrated so that every time the client's theta amplitude is greater than a level set by the therapist, the sound is heard. The sound suppresses the theta amplitude below the set threshold, so the sound turns off until the next time the theta amplitude rises above the threshold. This process usually continues for a short period of time, and then the client returns to regular neurofeedback therapy. The Braindryvr system for nudging the brain can help speed up the neurotherapy.

The Braindryvr system can also use LEDs to stimulate the brain whenever specific brainwave amplitudes are detected. For example, the system can be set up so that the LEDs stimulate at some fixed frequency, such as 15 Hz, whenever the client's theta amplitude rises above a specific threshold. The flashing LEDs have the effect of suppressing theta waves. In my clinic we often combine the theta-suppressing auditory harmonic and the theta-suppressing flashing lights when a client is engaged in a cognitive task. For example, if a child has a reading problem, the child reads during the theta-suppression treatment. This is an effective method for enhancing reading efficiency.

This brain-nudging system works well because the patient can exert control over the process. A child, for example, can focus her attention on keeping the harmonic tone off. I explain that when she does keep it off, the amplitude, or strength, of the brainwave band being trained is below the limit. When the tone goes on, it also contains a harmonic that suppresses the brainwave amplitude. Thus, the tone not only signals the need to concentrate but also assists the client by suppressing the brainwave amplitude.

With a few exceptions, brain-nudging systems are not generally used as the only form of neurotherapeutic treatment. The nudging systems are used briefly at various times during treatment to assist the regular neurofeedback treatment. The exceptions are when clients are not capable of participating effectively in a neurofeedback session. Some autistic children, for example, respond best to brain-driving procedures and may require prolonged use of a driver until they can participate in neurofeedback. Initially, autistic children may be incapable of attending to the game icons moving around the computer monitor. They are distracted, focused on pulling off the electrodes, and unresponsive to the treatment

provider's guidance and instructions. As brain activity starts to normalize as a result of the braindriving, the child becomes increasingly aware
of the treatment setting, the instructions of the therapist, and the video-
game figures on the monitor. At that time the child begins to become
capable of doing neurofeedback. Similarly, severely brain-injured clients
may not initially be capable of controlling the neurofeedback. In such
cases, brain-driving techniques are used as the major treatment method,
until the client eventually gains sufficient awareness to be treated with neurofeedback. Many manufacturers of neurofeedback equipment are now
incorporating brain-driving capabilities into the systems. These capabilities
permit the neurotherapist to use light and sound stimulation in the same
manner as that described above with the stand-alone Braindryvr unit.

## Other Supportive Treatments

Certain treatments are used to accelerate, synergize, and sustain neurotherapy. Brainwave activity can be modified in many ways. When you
concentrate, your brainwave activity changes. When you close your
eyes and imagine a ship sailing on the sea, slow brainwave amplitudes
increase in the back of the brain. If you focus on a light flashing at 12 Hz,
the brain usually produces increased brainwave amplitude around 12 Hz.
Sounds at specific frequencies, acupuncture stimulation, meditation, and
so on all have effects on brainwave activity. In this section we closely
examine a variety of treatment techniques and systems.

### Audiovisual Stimulation (AVS)

In the mid-1980s, when at the University of Ottawa, I conducted
research on the "flicker-fusion threshold." When you look at a flashing
light, either with eyes open in dim light or with eyes closed in bright
light, at a certain light-flash frequency you see the light as constant and
not as a flashing pulse. Some conditions, such as anxiety, may raise the
threshold at which the person no longer perceives the flashing. I was a university professor at the time and had a limited private practice. I treated
clients with anxiety-related problems such as headaches, irritable bowel
syndrome, sleep disturbances, and depression. When doing the research,
which used large strobe lights, I found that with eyes closed and at low

brightness, some frequencies were pleasant and relaxing. My patients reported relief from their symptoms when exposed to these low-frequency flashing lights. I also discovered that this procedure was used by hypnotists to relax clients as part of inducing them into a trance.

Today we do not use bulky research strobe lights but rather LEDs, which are attached to eyeglass frames, as described above. These LEDs come in a variety of colors because different visible wave lengths create different perceptions and sensations. Many companies manufacture these devices and call them by a variety of names, including light and sound machines and audiovisual stimulators. They are generally used for relaxing and invigorating the brain, as well as for nudging it, as described earlier. As noted above, when a person looks at a flashing light, the brainwave amplitude of that frequency usually increases. The beneficial effect of AVS is that it increases the strength of specific brainwave bands. If alpha amplitude is increased, for example, a sense of relaxation or calm increases.

AVS can be useful in treatment in several ways. Doil Montgomery of Nova Southeastern University and his colleagues have shown that visually stimulating subjects at 50 percent above or below their peak brainwave frequency will increase or decrease the peak frequency, respectively.[5] Increasing the peak frequency in the alpha band can have important benefits for one's general health and well-being. Home treatment with visual stimulators can be an efficient method for sustaining the gains of neurotherapy in maintaining a fast alpha peak frequency.

Neurotherapists often use AVS to supplement neurotherapy in the treatment of attention problems, learning problems, and autistic spectrum disorders. The AVS is used both in the office during the neurotherapy treatment and at home to support and enhance gains made during neurotherapy. For those concerned about photostrobic seizures, I would point out that these programs minimize the risk of having such a seizure. Photosensitive seizures, although rare, are typically associated with fixed or slowly changing flash frequency. The program I and many other neurotherapists use stimulates randomly between 10 and 18 Hz, changing every one to four seconds. This stimulation program is used with children with attention problems or specific learning problems such as reading, writing, spelling, and doing arithmetic. Special LED glasses that permit children to see through them allow the children to read or do other tasks while the brain is being stimulated.

Two special AVS programs have been developed, one for calming the brain and the other for a general brain "workout." The calming program randomly stimulates between 4 and 10 Hz, and the general workout program randomly stimulates between 5 and 24 Hz. In simple terms, the calming program is used before and immediately after a neurotherapy treatment focused on increasing slow brainwave amplitudes. The brain workout is typically used with seniors who complain of short-term memory problems. When the glasses are worn while reading, the workout program decreases slow-frequency amplitude, increases fast frequencies, and speeds up the alpha brainwaves. The person experiences increased focus and retention of information, and over time these brainwave changes become increasingly stable. Thus, for example, an elderly person who has had some memory problems associated with slowing alpha frequency will experience memory improvements. Further, because her reading may now be more efficient than in the past, she is likely to read more frequently, thereby exercising the brain and further improving her memory in a positively reinforcing cycle.

### Cranial Microamperage Stimulation (CES)

Cranial microamperage stimulation (CES) produces a low-amperage (always less than one milliampere) signal that is used to stimulate brain activity. At such a low amplitude, the technology is safe and effective. The frequency of the stimulation is between 0.3 and 100 Hz. Electrodes are placed at various locations about the head—on the bump directly behind each ear, on the forehead, at the back of the head, and on the earlobes. Most CES units have electrodes that attach to the earlobes like a clip-on earring. The units give stimulation that is set below the threshold of feeling and usually have automatic shut-offs to end the stimulation after a period of time, generally between twenty minutes and an hour.

CES technology was developed originally as a way to treat sleep problems. Electrosleep was one name used to describe this technology, which evolved from research in electromedicine in Russia and Eastern European countries, where the medical profession was less pharmaceutically dominated than in the United States. This technology has been rigorously tested and is now an FDA-registered medical treatment in the United States, where the purchase of a CES unit requires a prescription from a licensed health care provider. In Canada and many other countries, CES units are sold over-the-counter.

Considerable research has documented the effectiveness of CES technology in the treatment of many disorders, primarily those related to anxiety, depression, and substance abuse. Studies originally conducted for the FDA in 1995 and 1998 by Electromedical Products International, a manufacturer of one FDA-registered CES device, found that side effects of CES use were rare, and when they did occur, they were mild and self-limiting. Of nearly five hundred patients, 94 percent reported no side effects at all. Of the remaining 6 percent, most reported effects that were associated with setting the stimulation too high, and fewer than 1 percent reported skin irritation at the electrode site.[6] Ray Smith published, in 2001, the results of a survey of twenty-five hundred clients who used the CES device for pain management. Of the respondents, 93 percent reported more than 25 percent reduction in pain of all types. In addition, 90 percent reported reduced depression, 93 percent reported improved sleep, 94 percent reported less chronic fatigue, and 90 percent reported at least a 25 percent lessening of their anxiety.[7] All without drugs! In a study from the University of North Texas, Richard Kennerly reports that one of the effects of a twenty-minute CES session is a significant increase in alpha amplitude, which corresponds to users' reports of decreased anxiety after a CES treatment.[8]

CES can have several other effects on brainwave activity, such as increasing slow-frequency amplitude in the back of the brain. CES units help people with chronic pain, sleep problems, anxiety, depression, and addictions. For example, a typical treatment for a genetically predisposed alcoholic is the use of neurotherapy to increase theta amplitude in the back of the brain. As an adjunct to this treatment, neurotherapists often prescribe the daily use of a CES unit to help the alcoholic maintain sobriety by calming the central nervous system.

**FREQUENTLY ASKED QUESTION**

Q: I am feeling depressed, and my doctor suggested a trial of a mild antidepressant. Should I try it before considering neurotherapy?

A: You should consider doing neurotherapy first and avoid any entanglement with medications. Neurotherapy should be a first-choice primary-care treatment for mild depression.

In my clinic I use CES technology for adults only but not because I consider CES unsafe. Rather, I want to minimize the impact of the treatment on children's perception of their disorder and on their self-esteem. For example, many children do not want to take their prescribed Ritalin or other medication in school because they are embarrassed and feel less competent than children who do not require medication. I tell these children to think of their neurotherapy as a learning experience. Anything that we do in treatment is always presented as helping them gain control of their own brainwave activity. CES, like medications, can create a counterproductive mental attitude about the treatment because the electrodes make children feel strange. For this reason CES can reduce the efficiency of neurotherapy in children and thereby increase the number of treatment sessions required.

### Somatosensory Stimulation

Somatosensory stimulation is stimulation of the skin surfaces of the body. The stimulation can take many forms, including electricity, touch, needles, or magnets. CES technology can be extended to other areas of the body besides the ear lobes. Acupuncturists, for example, can use electrical stimulation rather than needles. A method called electroacustimulation (electro-acu-stimulation) is used in Chinese medicine to stimulate the body's energy. In 1993, I studied acupuncture at an institute affiliated with a psychiatric hospital in Shanghai, China. Although most people think of acupuncture as sticking needles into the body at various locations, these specific spots, or meridians, can be stimulated with pressure and electricity as well as with needles. According to Chinese medicine, the meridians are located along channels of energy in the body that, in turn, are attached to various organs. By stimulating the appropriate points, the therapist can treat problems associated with the attached organs. "Attached" may be the wrong word because these energy channels cannot be seen or measured with conventional measurement devices. However, they are measurable electrically. Scientist Chang-Li Zhang of the College of Life Sciences at Zhejiang University in China reports that the electrical resistance of the skin at acupuncture points is different from the resistance of the surrounding skin. These differences are reliable and allow tracking of the acupuncture meridian.[9]

In addition to the specific acupuncture meridians based on concepts of body-energy balance in traditional Chinese medicine (TCM), I was

taught that some points were chosen for the treatment of "mental problems" simply because they worked. I analyzed brainwave patterns associated with electrostimulation at several acupuncture points based on
what I had been taught by the TCM physicians in Shanghai. These points
included a meridian behind the ear, which I had already used with CES.
Used by acupuncturists to calm the client, stimulation of this meridian
increases slow-brainwave amplitude. Thus, a technique grounded in
conventional Western medicine corroborates what Chinese healers have
known for centuries.

Two other points have demonstrated effects on brainwave activity.
Pericardium 6 (P6) is located on the palm side of each forearm about
three finger widths above the crease at the wrist. Stimulation of this
point increases slow-brainwave amplitude and likewise has a calming
effect on the client. I use this stimulation point whenever nervous-
system hyperarousal is a problem. The P6 points are stimulated while
the client is receiving neurotherapy. P6 stimulation is frequently used to
help alcoholics and clients with seizure disorders. The second point is on
the Governor channel (Du26), located on the upper lip directly under
the nose. It was described to me as the "emergency" point for treatment
of clients with acute physical or mental symptoms. Stimulation of Du26
results in an immediate drop in slow-brainwave amplitude.

### Energy-Psychology Techniques
Acupuncture points are also stimulated manually using pressure,
rubbing, or tapping. Two unconventional procedures, Thought Field
Therapy (TFT) and the Emotional Freedom Technique (EFT), make use
of various combinations of acupuncture points that are stimulated in
sequence. Some of these procedures include whistling, moving the eyes
in particular ways, and standing in rather contorted positions prior to or
during the stimulation of the points. When I was first exposed to these
techniques at a conference in 2002, I dismissed them as bogus procedures that gained whatever benefit clients reported from placebo effects
and the charisma of the energy therapist. However, favorable reports
from several clients who had received such energy treatments encouraged me to look at the effects on brainwave activity.

The procedure I selected to study was EFT. To my knowledge at the
time, EFT was used primarily to treat phobias and other anxiety-based

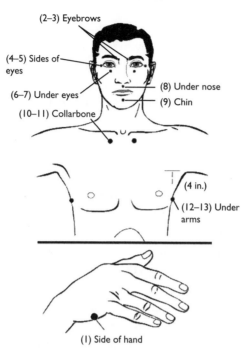

*Figure 5. Tapping points for self-administration of the EFT. Numbers indicate the sequence.*

disorders. This technique involves tapping thirteen acupuncture points in sequence. It also includes a self-affirmation while tapping the first meridian, which is "Even though I have [the problem], I deeply and completely accept myself." The points and the sequence in which they are tapped are shown in Figure 5. After the affirmation, one taps each meridian three or four times while thinking about the problem. The entire sequence can be done in about ten seconds. For example, if you were afraid of elevators, you would say while tapping the point on the hand, "Even though I am afraid to ride elevators, I deeply and completely accept myself." Then you would proceed to the inner edge of the eyebrow and would tap each location in sequence three or four times while repeating the word "elevators" or thinking about elevators.

Skeptical? I certainly was. However, after reviewing some research on these techniques, I realized that this method of using the acupuncture energy system warranted serious consideration. Several studies had indicated that, at least at the subjective level, these techniques benefited clients. I attended a conference where practitioners of these techniques described cases in which clients reported major improvements with various phobias and anxiety-related conditions. The entire October 2001 issue of the *Journal of Clinical Psychology* was devoted to research and commentary on TFT. The studies demonstrated major positive changes in heart-rate variability (HRV) with TFT treatments. HRV is an important indicator of health that is relatively unaffected by most treatments and placebo effects. Lee Pulos, Mari Swingle, and I studied the effects of EFT on clients with PTSD following motor-vehicle accidents. We found that the brainwave indicators of anxiety and depressed mood improved substantially after EFT treatments.[10]

Given the reports of favorable improvements in phobic reactions of clients, I was curious about the effects of EFT on SMR, an important brainwave indicator of body quiet (see Chapter 2). I examined the brainwave activity of clients before and after doing an EFT sequence and found that SMR increased immediately. You may recall that SMR enhancement is the primary neurotherapeutic treatment for seizure disorders. Thus, I tried using EFT as a supplementary home treatment while the client received SMR neurofeedback treatment for epilepsy. The results were astonishing. The SMR treatment for seizure disorder can require many sessions, typically in the range of fifty to eighty. With the help of EFT, successful seizure remission and reduction has been accomplished in as few as twelve sessions.[11]

**FREQUENTLY ASKED QUESTION**

Q: My wife is pregnant and has a serious sleep problem. Her doctor prescribed a sleeping medication he said was safe for pregnant women. My wife does not want to take any medications during her pregnancy, but she is really suffering from not sleeping. Are there safe medications?
A: I agree with your wife—she should avoid drugs during pregnancy. Psychologists have many good treatments for sleep-quality problems, one of which is neurotherapy. Find a qualified neurotherapist or psychologist with experience in treating sleep disturbance.

One client, upon learning that she was pregnant, wanted to eliminate or strongly reduce her antiseizure medication. Sarah was aware of the recent finding that antiseizure medications previously considered safe result in an increased frequency of learning disorders, particularly in male children. Using EFT, she had an unprecedented increase in SMR amplitude, and within four visits she was free of seizures on half the medication. After seven sessions she stopped taking the medication entirely.

Another success story was that of Glen, a thirteen-year-old patient. At the initial assessment, his theta/SMR ratio was high. For the two months prior to treatment he had been having "staring spells" three to four times per week. His major seizures had been fairly well controlled by a ketogenic diet, which features a heavy fat intake, but the goal was to take Glen totally off antiseizure medication and the special diet. Glen was taught the EFT method, and by the fourth neurofeedback session his theta/SMR ratio was reduced by almost half. The theta/SMR ratio is the ratio of the electrical amplitude, measured in microvolts, of brainwave bands 3–7 Hz divided by 13–15 Hz. This ratio is associated with seizures, and reductions in this ratio are related to reduction in seizure activity.[12] After seven sessions Glen's mother reported greatly improved cognitive functioning and improved relationships with his peers. His theta/SMR ratio was finally reduced to a third and has remained stable at between 2.0 and 2.5. He is presently on a maintenance schedule of neurofeedback every two months; his grateful mother left the following voice mail: "Hi, Dr. Swingle, this is Claire calling. I have been bringing my son Glen to see you now since March, and I just wanted to pass on some very good news. . . . We went for an EEG yesterday and for the first time in eight years . . . our EEG actually showed quite significant improvement. He's always had a bad EEG. Now he is getting a fairly good EEG, and he got an excellent report from the psychologist as well, so I just wanted to pass on the news to you."[13]

### Neuroactive Harmonics

The supplementary treatment that most profoundly enhances neurofeedback is neuroactive auditory harmonics. These were developed quite by accident. One day in my laboratories at Ottawa University, I was trying to perfect a sound signal for use on a relaxation tape. Basically, the sound was like the rise and fall in pitch associated with a siren. While I was working, one of my graduate students came over and complained that he had been overcome by fatigue. It was only 8:30 in the morning, and he said that he had felt fine until a short time before, when he had become very sleepy. He further reported that he had slept well the previous night and was in a refreshed and alert state when he arrived at his office, which was located in my laboratories about thirty feet from where I was working. While pondering this dilemma, we realized that the sound I was working with, although clearly audible to me, was below the hearing threshold in the student's office. We checked this theory out, and indeed the sound was subliminal there. Although I had been involved in research focused on the clinical effects of verbal subliminal messages and had published my book *Subliminal Treatment Procedures: A Clinician's Guide,* which summarized ten years of research, this event triggered further investigation of the use of blended subliminal harmonic sounds as supplementary treatments in neurotherapy.

Subliminal sound is presented below the threshold for hearing. However, even though you cannot hear the sound, the sound can affect your mood, thoughts, and physiological functions. The sound has to be kept within a critical range otherwise there are no measurable effects. Sound within the critical range can have a marked effect on brainwave activity such as slow-frequency (theta) amplitude. We now have neuroactive harmonics that affect several brainwave bandwidths. They are used in the treatment of all attention and learning disorders, as well as many anxiety-based disorders. The specific sound that fatigued my graduate student was refined and is now used to enhance sleep. Another time, I was listening to a recently recorded harmonic designed to induce nausea in order to assess the quality of the recording. A family member came in from an adjoining room and said she suddenly felt nauseous, not knowing the harmonic was playing. This "aversion" harmonic is now used in conjunction with neurotherapy in the treatment of addictions.

The most important harmonic is used to treat attention deficiencies that are associated with excessive slow-brainwave amplitudes. This harmonic, which I call Alert, has an immediate effect on theta amplitude measured at the top of the head. As we have already discussed, many forms of ADD are associated with excessive theta brainwaves, and the goal of neurotherapy is to reduce them. Research conducted on college students, adults with ADD, children with ADD and ADHD, and clients with mild TBI demonstrated a robust and consistent suppression of theta amplitude with this harmonic.[14] After more than ten years of use, thousands of clients have been treated with Alert.

The procedure is straightforward. During the initial assessment, the effect of Alert on a patient's theta amplitude is measured directly. If the harmonic suppresses theta waves, which it does in over 90 percent of clients with attention problems, Alert is prescribed for home use. Clients simply play the Alert harmonic, which is recorded on CD, while reading, doing homework, or engaging in some other cognitively challenging activity. The harmonic sounds like pink noise—just a "shush" sound, a bit like running water—and it is specifically designed to be most effective at very low volume, so it does not interfere at all with doing homework. Use of the Alert harmonic for just fifteen minutes per day can reduce the number of neurotherapy sessions from the forty to sixty previously required to less than half that number. My favorite testimonial came from a teacher in a school where the Alert harmonic was used to help students concentrate. The teacher wrote, "Our problem was that we originally only ordered two [Alert] tapes. The teachers who had the most immediate and dramatic results with their students would not lend their tapes [to] the rest of the staff."

Another harmonic frequently used in neurofeedback has the reverse effect. This harmonic, called Serene, reduces fast brainwave activity or increases slow activity or both. This harmonic is used with clients who would benefit from additional calming of the central nervous system while they are undergoing neurofeedback treatment. The harmonic also helps in treating sleep disturbances.

One reason harmonics work so well is that the effects on the client are evaluated in the clinic. As mentioned, during the initial brain mapping, clients are exposed to the harmonic thought to be appropriate for their treatment, and any change in brainwave activity is determined. If the harmonic does not change brainwave activity in the desired manner, that harmonic is not prescribed for the client. Thus, we know exactly how the harmonic is going to work before it is prescribed for home use.

The harmonics are available through many websites. Two major sites are Soundhealthproducts.com (which offers directly downloadable files in addition to CDs) and Toolsforwellness.com. Most neurotherapists use or are familiar with these products as they are described in many of the treatment manuals written for clinicians.

### Peripheral Biofeedback

An important treatment often used in conjunction with neurotherapy is peripheral biofeedback. One of the fundamental techniques used in neurotherapy, brainwave biofeedback is feedback of brain activity that controls the central nervous system. Peripheral biofeedback, in contrast, is usually focused on the activity of the autonomic nervous system (ANS). The ANS is divided into two major components, the sympathetic nervous system (SNS) and the parasympathetic nervous system (PNS). All the organs in the body are connected to the ANS. The two divisions may be likened to the accelerator and the brakes on an automobile. Although this analogy is oversimplified, the SNS supplies arousal and preparation for fight or flight. The PNS controls body calming and recovery. The SNS generally raises levels of activation, whereas the PNS lowers levels of activation. If your heart speeds up too much, for example, the PNS slows it down. Conversely, if your heart slows excessively, the SNS speeds it up. Some organs are regulated by only one branch of the ANS. Blood flow at the skin surface of your feet, for example, is controlled only by the SNS. Peripheral ANS biofeedback modifies the activity of the PNS and the SNS. Animals, including chimpanzees and cats, can be taught to modify brainwave activity. Edward Taub, when at the University of Alabama in 1998, reported on a study showing that adult male monkeys could reduce muscle tension in the forearm of the dominant arm by an average of 50 percent over a ten-session training period.[15] Animal subjects prove that brainwave control works because animals do not respond to placebo, the expectation of an outcome. Animal research shows that these techniques can also modify the peripheral nervous system independent of the subjects' thought system.

Electromyographic (EMG) biofeedback provides you with information on the tension of your muscles, as measured by electrical activity. You can use this direct feedback to learn how to relax muscle tension. EMG biofeedback is valuable in the treatment of motor disorders in clients who have TBI or have had a stroke. It also eases muscle-pain problems, including lower-back pain and headaches. Neurotherapists also frequently use EMG feedback of the muscles of the forehead as a general relaxation treatment.

I met Harry when I was coordinator of the psychophysiology service at McLean Hospital in Belmont, Massachusetts. Harry had been hospitalized because he was suicidally depressed. For the previous five years, he had suffered from a condition that started as a persistent headache and subsequently was experienced as a feeling of pressure and profound cognitive "fuzziness." He was in continuous discomfort, could not think properly, and had lost his job. He became increasingly withdrawn from friends and family and experienced frequent and intense episodes of depression with strong suicidal fantasies.

During Harry's many hospitalizations, numerous diagnostic tests had failed to identify the cause of his problem. He was referred to me to determine whether neurotherapy might help. Yet the various brain scans did not show anything extraordinary. The nature of Harry's symptoms suggested instead that the peripheral autonomic nervous system, rather than the central nervous system (the brain), should be examined. The peripheral systems include muscles, the vascular system, heart functions, skin response, and breathing. To test Harry, his muscle tension, peripheral blood flow (usually measured by skin-surface temperature), electrodermal response (electrical resistance of the skin), heart rate, and breathing were measured both at rest and when he was exposed to a minor stressor. The stressor that I generally use is having the client count backward by sevens from some arbitrary number such as 713. The counting is done out loud. This procedure increases heart rate, blood pressure, and other indicators of peripheral neural function. This assessment provides a lot of information about the ANS's level of arousal. At rest, the muscle tension in Harry's forehead was 7.8 microvolts, and it increased to 12.8 microvolts when he was counting backward. The tension in the forehead should be around 2 microvolts, and when the client is counting, the increase should be in the range of 1.5 microvolts. Harry's other measurements indicated normal levels and normal reactions to stress.

It seemed likely that Harry's problem was caused by excessive tension in the muscles of the head. To test this assumption, I had Harry do muscle biofeedback of the muscles in the head and also of the muscles of his upper torso. Harry was able to substantially reduce the muscle tension in his forehead in a short time. As the muscle tension decreased, Harry's electrodermal response increased remarkably. Electrodermal activity responds to emotional feelings. When you have an emotional thought, electrodermal activity usually shows a rapid jump as sweat glands are activated. We all have this experience when we have an intense reaction such as fear and we become sweaty or "clammy." In Harry's case, electrodermal activity occurred when he started to cry. I asked him about his crying, and he told me, "The pressure in my head is gone." I explained to Harry that his problem was essentially a tension head-ache. Because he experienced this discomfort as pressure and "fuzziness" in the head rather than head pain, the tension headache was not diagnosed. Further, because his depression was a reaction to the pain and not neuro-logically based, antidepressant medication was largely ineffective.

Harry's treatment consisted of a few sessions of muscle biofeedback to teach him how to recognize when his muscles were tense and how to relax them. I also taught Harry some muscle-relaxation exercises for home use. In addition, he needed psychological therapy and counselling to help him plan his reentry into social and work environments. Treating Harry's problem directly with muscle relaxation was clearly the most effective treatment. Harry, incidentally, was angry with his former "experts." He checked himself out of the hospital immediately after his assessment and first treatment session with me and had some unkind words for the physician who had hospitalized him several times over the previous months. Harry's response to the muscle-tension biofeedback was nothing short of miraculous. It is extraordinarily unusual for a client to respond so rapidly. Normally it would require many sessions for a client to reduce the tension to a level at which a beneficial change in the symptom would be reported.

For muscle-tension problems such as headaches, home treatment can be helpful. The home EMG units require that the client attach stick-on electrodes to the affected area, such as the forehead. Wires from these electrodes feed into the EMG monitoring device, which gives visual and auditory feedback about the tension in the muscle. The client uses that feedback to learn how to reduce the tension. This is a standard treatment for certain forms of headache and nighttime bruxism (teeth grinding).

Peripheral blood flow is the blood volume in the arterioles and venules (small arteries and veins) near the surface of your skin. Cold hands are the result of a reduction in your peripheral blood flow. Blood flow can be measured in several ways, including by the pulse blood volume or, more generally, by surface body temperature. As blood flow increases, surface body temperature increases. Blood flow and temperature biofeedback are effective treatment methods. One terrific method for enhancing body relaxation is hand-warming biofeedback. In the study described earlier, Taub showed that monkeys can change their hand temperature. The monkeys were first trained to increase hand temperature. After twenty-five sessions hand temperature increased by an average of 1.8°F. The monkeys were then taught to lower hand temperature. After twenty-five sessions hand temperature dropped 1.8° and an additional 0.7° below the animals' original starting temperature. (In clinical practice, therapists have found that it is more difficult for clients to lower hand temperature than to raise it.)

Setting up hand-warming biofeedback is simple. The skin-surface transducers are very sensitive, so minute changes are measured, and the feedback is rapid. Clients can see the immediate results of their efforts to change hand temperature. Through trial and error they soon learn how to focus attention on their hands, and they experience a gradual sensation of warmth. A feeling of calm accompanies increasing hand warmth. As your body relaxes, your hands warm, and, conversely, as you warm your hands, feelings of calm and serenity usually follow.

Hand warming is often used as a first step in many neurotherapy treatments. For example, clients with severe anxiety are treated with brainwave biofeedback to increase the amplitude of theta in the back of the brain. This treatment can often be speeded up if the client is first trained to increase hand temperature and experiences its relaxing effect. Hand warming is often used prior to neurotherapy in the treatment of some forms of alcoholism as well. The client is first taught to increase hand temperature to calm the ANS. After several successful sessions, neurofeedback of slow-wave activity in the back of the brain starts. Thermal biofeedback is also effective in treating vascular disorders such as migraine headaches, Raynaud's disease, and hypertension. It can also be used to treat some sleep disorders, such as nocturnal myoclonus (jerking leg movements), which is related to reduced blood flow in the legs and feet.

Electrodermal biofeedback is another useful treatment. As noted above, when you become aroused (for example, by thinking about something exciting or being startled by a loud noise), the electrical resistance of your skin drops as sweat glands are activated. The skin is a remarkably responsive organ and reflects subtle changes in emotions and sympathetic and parasympathetic stimulation such as abrupt changes in breathing. Frequently used to help relaxation, the electrodermal response (EDR) can be a remarkably sensitive indicator of the emotional significance of thoughts, ideas, and memories. In psychotherapy sessions, the EDR is used to indicate the emotional significance of the issues being discussed. Often the full emotional significance of a conscious thought is not obvious to the client. The EDR in such cases can reveal latent emotional dispositions that need to be discussed during therapy.

Biofeedback treatment can be used in conjunction with neurotherapy to address many other medical issues, including problems with heart rate, heart rhythm, blood pressure, blood pulse volume, respiration rate, pupil dilation, and voice characteristics. Some of the treatments can be administered at home with the use of portable units. The home-training units are usually easy to use. A familiar example is the heart-rate monitor you may be using as part of your exercise programs. Some of these monitors have alarms that warn you if the heart is beating too quickly, so you can slow down the exercise pace. The biofeedback monitors work on much the same principle, but have higher levels of precision and accuracy, give continuous feedback, and usually provide more detailed information. A treatment heart monitor might, for example, also provide feedback information on heart rhythm, irregular beats, and the blood volume of each beat in addition to beat frequency. Many common biofeedback treatments, such as those that correct muscle tension, skin conductance, heart rate, and skin temperature, can be readily supplemented with home units. In some cases, most of the treatment, such as EMG training for a simple tension headache, can be done at home. For others, such as back pain, the amount of home treatment is minimal.

Other problems require office treatments. Measurement of respiration and the volume of air intake with each breath requires an apparatus too cumbersome for home use. This form of air-flow or respiration-rate treatment is often warranted for breathing problems, asthma, and panic disorders. The measurement of voice characteristics requires a sound-controlled environment, and measuring pupil size requires head restraints and elaborate measurement equipment. Also, some treatments require office visits because of the complexity of the procedures. In treating lower-back pain, many EMG electrodes are placed at several locations on the back. The client is guided through specific moves to learn to tense and relax various muscle groups in precise sequence to correct the back problem.

**FREQUENTLY ASKED QUESTION**

Q: My seventy-nine-year-old mother seems very depressed. She says it's just that she's growing old. She won't take any medication for depression, but she does take a sleeping pill. Would neurotherapy help?

A: Neurotherapy could help significantly with the sleep disturbance and the depression. In addition, I would recommend some behavioral counseling to help your mother revitalize her interests.

## Additional Levels of Neurotherapy: Preventative Maintenance and Optimal-Performance Training

The brain, being a dynamic organ, becomes increasingly efficient and intellectually expansive when it is functioning optimally. Hence, maintaining the brain with periodic "tune-ups" not only sustains efficient functioning but facilitates continued intellectual growth and development. We often see our senior clients about four times per year to "brighten" the brain. Treatment usually involves increasing the speed of the peak alpha frequencies, a procedure that delays age-related intellectual decline. For younger clients, two or so visits per year are usually adequate as a maintenance program.

Maintenance biofeedback for the brain may have far-reaching effects on health and well-being. As discussed in Chapter 3, Michael Doppelmayr and Wolfgang Klimesch at the University of Salzburg in Austria have shown that the strength of alpha brainwaves is directly associated with cognitive performance. The dominant frequency of the alpha band is likewise important, with faster frequencies being associated with better cognitive performance. In addition, robust alpha strength, frequency, and efficiency (that is, how quickly the strength of alpha signals changes under different task demands) have been shown to be related to general health and well-being. People with fast peak alpha frequency, for example, are healthier than individuals having lower frequencies. The balance of the alpha amplitude between the right and the left frontal brain regions is also important. Imbalances can be related to several conditions including depression and fatigue. Alpha variables have also been shown to be related to schizophrenia, dementias, emotional states, anxiety, stroke recovery, cerebral blood flow, and brain oxygenation. In short, keeping one's alpha "healthy" appears to be good preventative medicine.

**FREQUENTLY ASKED QUESTION**

Q: My psychologist told me that neurotherapy doesn't last and that you have to keep going for more treatments. Is this true?

A: With the exception of a few age-related neurological changes that require periodic treatment, once a problem is remedied, it remains in this improved state without further sessions.

The alpha maintenance program may seem at odds with my statement that "once it's fixed, it's fixed." This statement refers to normalizing brainwave activity so that symptoms associated with dysfunction can be eliminated. In this sense once the brainwave activity has been normalized, it is, indeed, "fixed." However, as with any other bodily system, changes may occur with illness and with aging. Keeping the alpha peak frequency fast with neurotherapy can help ameliorate or slow down the progressive, age-related effects of the alpha slowing.

Another level of neurotherapy is optimal-performance, or peak-performance, training. If you want to be physically fit, you might visit the gym three or four times each week. For peak athletic performance, however, additional work is required. A person who wants to compete at championship, Olympic, or professional levels spends hours each day in the gym. Likewise with optimal brain functioning, keeping the brain in the upper ranges of functioning requires systematic and frequent training sessions.

Russell Adams, writing in the July 29, 2006, issue of the *Wall Street Journal,* describes how months before the World Cup soccer playoffs, some of Italy's best players began spending much of their practice time doing neurofeedback. Italy won the World Cup, and the team referred to the neurofeedback as their secret weapon. In the same article, Adams describes optimal-performance neurotherapy training with a high school football player who went on to play for Boston College. Rae Tattenbaum, from Hartford, Connecticut, provided the neurotherapy training for this young man, and she informed me that every night he listened to the Alert harmonic to increase his focus. The Alert harmonic, described previously in this chapter, is used routinely with clients with ADHD to help them with focus.

Sometimes neurotherapy that is focused on optimizing a brain function brings to the surface a memory or emotional state that the client must resolve before moving on. This is not a problem but rather one of the side benefits of brainwave therapy. Potent memories and emotional states can interfere with your quality of life even though you are not fully aware of them. Unexplained difficulties in intimate relationships are a common result of poorly perceived personal problems. Resolving these problems can have marked benefit for the client's well-being.


## Home Treatment

With the development of relatively low-cost devices for brainwave biofeedback, clients occasionally inquire about the possibility of treating themselves or their children at home. When considering self-treatment, you should keep in mind that neurofeedback is not a stand-alone therapy. A widely held notion is that all a therapist needs to do to treat depression, for example, is to place EEG sensors over the left frontal lobe and tell the client to "increase the amplitude of beta." It is true that beta enhancement generally helps in treating depression, but it is never adequate as a sole treatment. Some form of additional cognitive therapy or behavioral therapy or both is always required. The combination makes for remarkably rapid, efficient, and lasting treatment. Indeed, the treatment of any disorder rarely, if ever, involves only one method. Treatment requires work at various sites on the brain to modify brain activity that may be exacerbating the condition.

Learning to correct brain functioning is, in some ways, similar to using a personal coach in physical training. One of the major functions of the neurotherapist is to help the client learn to modify brain activity by a process called behavioral shaping. Shaping refers to gradually increasing the level of difficulty as the client becomes better at producing the response. Thus, I advise people not to engage in unsupervised neurofeedback at home unless they are training merely for relaxation or focus.

However, using home-based treatments under the supervision of a well-trained neurotherapist can be helpful. The newer equipment systems have been designed so that specific treatment protocols can be loaded into the unit for home use. The results of each treatment session are retained in the unit. The therapist can then analyze and modify the method as treatment progresses. Some systems now available are linked to a central computer in the therapist's office; the therapist can directly monitor each session the client is receiving at home, making changes as needed.

The level of monitoring required for treatment at a satellite location may be substantial, and so the savings over office-based treatment may not be much. However, if a single protocol is to be used for many sessions, then the home-based treatment can be quite economical. In the treatment of some forms of ADD, for example, a number of sessions focus on the suppression of slow-wave amplitudes over a specific region in the brain. Home-based sessions for this specific method are a good complement to in-office treatments.

A promising application of the remote systems is in schools. Technicians trained in neurotherapy can administer treatment protocols for students whose learning and attention difficulties have been assessed by a neurotherapist. Each session can be reviewed and modified as needed, and thus many students can receive economical treatment conveniently and under the direct supervision of a qualified neurotherapist. Several pilot projects provide evidence that school-based brainwave biofeedback can produce strong benefits. William Boyd and Susan Campbell reported on a pilot study of six students treated with neurotherapy in a Wyoming public school.[16] The students were all diagnosed with ADD and received, on average, twenty sessions of neurofeedback. The results indicated significant improvement in measures of attention and intelligence. In a larger study of sixteen children in a Yonkers, New York, elementary school, neurofeedback significantly improved the attention of ADHD students.[17] Unfortunately, many neurotherapists, those in my clinic included, who have tried to introduce neurotherapy into schools have met with bureaucratic resistance. I negotiated with one school for over a year, only to be ultimately refused. I also have been denied even a preliminary interview with school officials on the issue of neurotherapy in schools. The potential savings to school boards because of reduced special-needs service is sizable, but so far only progressive school officials have been taking the first steps toward what may become a nationwide method of helping special-needs children in school.

Finally, never treat yourself or any family member without close supervision. Curing a child through neurotherapy, even though it looks like game playing, is not like teaching him how to play Monopoly. Serious issues of judgment, motivation, objectivity, and singleness of purpose are involved. Because of family dynamics, a child's treatment may be seriously undercut by power struggles, feelings of disapproval, fear of failure, and lack of motivation. Further, a parent lacks the skill necessary to keep a sustained focus on treatment in all of its areas. Some systems designed for home use have exciting and engaging graphics to sustain the interest and compliance of the child. Yet compelling evidence indicates that these systems are largely ineffective in the treatment of problems such as AD(H)D. The child may be interested enough to use the system, but typically the attentional problems remain unchanged because no learning or brain changes have occurred. As most parents know, an ADD child can spend hours a day playing video games without any changes. In fact, many parents report that the problem gets worse the more hours that are spent at the computer terminal. Systems that focus on game playing rather than brain changes are simply going to sustain the ADD. In my experience, home-based treatments that are not directly supervised by a neurotherapist are inevitably abandoned at some point. The damage done to the children can be substantial because they may conclude both that neurotherapy is not effective and that they themselves are defective and incurable, a viewpoint likely to be shared by the parent.

The problems of family dynamics that frequently interfere with home-based treatments can be overcome. Problems can be minimized if someone other than the parent, such as a teacher or a college student, administers the treatment on a scheduled basis. Older children can, at times, administer their own treatment as directed by the neurotherapist. In such cases, the parent may help the child by attaching the electrodes and then leaving the child alone. After several in-office treatments, children can often learn the basics of the protocol and become quite capable of making necessary adjustments during a treatment session. In a family with loving parents, a mixture of parent-administered and child-administered sessions can work.

In summary, unless there are compelling reasons to consider home-based treatment, such as living a long distance from a neurotherapist, office-based treatment is decidedly the preferred method. Because issues other than the neurotherapy need to be addressed in the treatment of almost any disorder, office visits are far more effective and more likely to result in significant improvement than are home treatments.

There are many ways to modify brain functioning. Some of the methods described in this chapter have a temporary effect that is made stable with neurofeedback. Other treatments have a lasting effect on their own and serve to speed up the neurotherapy. In the next chapter we see how these procedures are used in the treatment of a variety of disorders. Some of these, such as a common form of ADD, are relatively simple problems that a few neurofeedback treatments plus the home use of a sub-threshold harmonic can resolve. Others are complex and require a variety of treatment techniques plus psychotherapy to be corrected.

CHAPTER 5

# Diagnostic Chaos: The Case of ADHD

In my experience, the diagnosis of brain-functioning disorders such as ADHD is chaotic in that the same label is attached to vastly different combinations of symptoms. Hence, from a clinical perspective, the label is useless for it carries no information that would help a neurotherapist decide on a regimen of treatment. As you may have noticed, I tend to avoid the use of diagnostic labels in this book (as well as in my clinic). I prefer to speak not of ADHD but rather of attention deficiencies. I avoid diagnostic labels not only because they are often useless but because the stigma attached to the label can have extremely negative consequences.

Entire industries have emerged that focus on putting labels on human physical and psychological complaints. A patient or student can be exposed to days of psychological testing. Once these Herculean efforts are completed, a label or labels are offered with various levels of opinionated certainty. The question I always ask after these ordeals are completed is, "Now what?" Do the labels have any therapeutic implications? Usually the answer to this question is no. The treatments pursued are going to be largely trial-and-error anyway. Conventional therapists likely will try medication A because it often is thought useful with a specific characteristic, such as hyperactivity. If the parents report favorable results, they stay with the treatment. If the reports from the parents are not positive, then the dosage is increased or a new medication is tried. Does this process sound familiar to you?

In addition, there is a bureaucratic answer to the question, Why are labels used for problematic behaviors? Many parents strongly resist labeling their children because of the potentially harmful effects of stigmatization and threats to self-esteem. However, they find that unless they allow the child to be labeled, assistance is unavailable. Without a diagnostic label the children are not eligible for special assistance programs in school, or for government financial assistance to pay for special tutors and behavioral programs, or for insurance coverage for treatment.

The philosophical basis for neurological brain mapping is different from the basis of the labeling process. Neurotherapists see a problem in brain functioning as a window of opportunity for correcting the problem. Health care providers tend to accept diagnostic labels as evidence of a chronic condition, with negative implications for the patient's expectation of a positive outcome. From a neurotherapeutic perspective, these problems can be corrected. They are not considered chronic disorders that, at best, can be managed with continuous treatment.

Nowhere is the contrast between neurotherapy and conventional medical intervention more evident than in the treatment of ADHD. In the first place, ADD and ADHD are useless labels from a therapeutic perspective. People use the terms as a shorthand in conversation: "My child has ADD," meaning she has problems in school that appear to be the result of her inability to sustain attention. "My child has ADHD," meaning he (more often male) is doing poorly in school, which appears to be the result of his not being able to sit still and focus, or he is being disruptive in the classroom or he is both doing poorly and is disruptive. These labels are simply general symptom descriptions and do not reliably identify an underlying categorical disorder.

Table 1, taken from the *Diagnostic and Statistical Manual of Mental Disorders,* lists behaviors that are considered indicators of ADHD. There is quite a wide range, and children can have any number of combinations of these characteristics. The ADD or ADHD label is applied if those assessing the child (for instance parents, teachers, psychiatrists) indicate that he displays these characteristics with a certain frequency or strength relative to the other children. The usual rule of thumb for a diagnosis of ADHD is that the child possesses at least six of the inattentive characteristics for over six months or, for the hyperactive form, the child possesses six or more of the hyperactive characteristics for over six months.

## TABLE I: DIAGNOSTIC CRITERIA FOR ADHD

Six or more of the following symptoms of inattention have persisted for at least six months to a degree that is maladaptive and inconsistent with developmental level:

*Inattention:*
Often fails to give close attention to details or makes careless mistakes in schoolwork, work, or other activities.

Often has difficulty sustaining attention in tasks or play activities.

Often does not seem to listen when spoken to directly.

Often does not follow through on instructions and often fails to finish schoolwork, chores, or duties in the workplace (not due to oppositional behavior or failure to understand instructions).

Often has difficulty organizing tasks and activities.

Often avoids, dislikes, or is reluctant to engage in tasks that require sustained mental effort (such as schoolwork or homework).

Often loses things necessary for tasks or activities (e.g., toys, school assignments, pencils, books, or tools).

Is often easily distracted by extraneous stimuli.

Is often forgetful in daily activities.

Six or more of the following symptoms of hyperactivity/impulsivity have persisted for at least six months to a degree that is maladaptive and inconsistent with developmental level:

*Hyperactivity:*
Often fidgets with hands or feet or squirms in seat.

Often leaves seat in classroom or in other situations in which remaining seated is expected.

Often runs about or climbs excessively in situations in which it is inappropriate (in adolescents or adults, may be limited to subjective feelings of restlessness).

Often has difficulty playing or engaging in leisure activities quietly.

Is often "on the go" or often acts as if "driven by a motor."

Often talks excessively.

*Impulsivity:*
Often blurts out answers before questions have been completed.

Often has difficulty awaiting turn.

Often interrupts, intrudes on others (e.g., butts into conversations or games).

Source: American Psychiatric Association, *Diagnostic and Statistical Manual of Mental Disorders*, 4th ed. (Washington, D.C.: American Psychiatric Association, 2007), 92.

Unfortunately, the checklist method of diagnosing a deficiency such as ADHD is extremely subjective and often tells more about the person making the assessment than about the child being assessed.

Alan's story is a case in point. The ten-year-old was making good progress in my sessions, changing his brainwave activity. In addition, he reported improvements in school and a modest improvement in grades. Yet one day he told me that his psychiatrist had increased his dosage of methylphenidate (Ritalin). Surprised, I asked his mother why. She said that although Alan's school-related behavior was improving (for example, he was finishing his homework more rapidly and completely and with far less prodding than before), his teacher had complained of continued problems. Alan was still talkative in class, and the teacher was annoyed. The psychiatrist had requested a checklist evaluation from Alan, the teacher, and the parents. Based on the teacher's response, the psychiatrist concluded that the ADHD had increased in severity, and she increased the dosage. Neither the parents' nor the child's checklist evaluations concurred with the teacher's assessment. The psychiatrist was medicating Alan because of the teacher's impatience or inability to tolerate ten-year-old behavior that may well have been within the normal range or that might have been managed through a coordinated in-class behavior program.

An increase in medication often has a negative effect on brainwave treatment, as it did in this case, because it discourages both the child and the parents. To evaluate this situation I administered an attention-assessment test, virtually the only standardized test that I use and then only infrequently. There are several such tests. They require the client to respond to a stimulus over and over again. For example, the test may require that the child press a key whenever a letter appears except when the letter X appears. The child is encouraged to press the key as rapidly as possible. Because the tests are repetitive and last for about fifteen minutes, they are boring, and all clients eventually lose focus, particularly those with an attention or a hyperactivity problem. The results of the test indicated that Alan had only one category of response that was statistically "mildly atypical"; there was no evidence of an attention difficulty. Based on the results of this test, the parents' subjective evaluation, and Alan's self-report, the parents gradually reduced the medication without informing the teacher or the psychiatrist. The parents and I also praised Alan for his excellent progress and counseled him about appropriate behavior in the classroom. (One can use many behavioral techniques with motivated children to help modify behavior in the classroom.)

---

**FREQUENTLY ASKED QUESTION**

Q: My son has ADHD and has serious problems at school. We put him on Ritalin, which has helped a lot, but I'm concerned about the negative effects of long-term use. What should we do?

A: Because of the risks, I would move quickly to treat the ADHD and get your son off the medication. Many parents have found that intensive neurotherapy during a drug-free vacation time is adequate for the child to return to school medication-free.

---

Some neurotherapists like to administer tests, usually computerized, of various cognitive abilities to quantify the improvements associated with the neurotherapy. In general, I have no quarrel with this idea. The data may be useful for research purposes, and therapists feel that they gain a degree of precision with frequent testing. My own preference is to rely on observable changes in brainwave activity. The reason I rely so heavily on the data obtained from the brain map is because the brain tells a complete story. Many conditions are associated with attention difficulties. The brainwave data suggest what the problem is, where it resides, and how to fix it. Psychological testing is an indirect method for assessing a problem that can be directly observed from the data supplied by the brain. More important, I rely on the client's own reports of progress. I ask my clients to maintain records of the symptoms they wish to modify. The changes in their self-reports then become an evaluation of changes resulting from the treatment.

The chaos associated with the diagnosis of ADHD is apparent in the wide array of books on the subject. This chaos seems inevitable because of the great many types of attention deficiencies. Further, many other conditions and disorders mimic ADHD. One theory of conflict is that people who attain positions of influence or power during crises are likely to sustain the conflict in order to retain their positions of influence. What would happen to the ADHD pundits if ADHD was cured? The books on the burdens of living with this disorder would be largely irrelevant. Ironically, many of the popular books on the subject of

ADHD have been written by people who claim to have survived and even prospered because of their ADHD.

One problem neurotherapists often encounter is that clients or parents of clients are pessimistic about brainwave treatment precisely because they have read one of these books. The message such books communicate is that ADD is an incurable chronic disorder that must be accepted and coped with by use of medications, family counseling, and special educational programs and privileges. Entire industries established to help clients and families cope with ADHD depend to a large extent on its being categorized as a chronic disorder. Because ADHD is considered chronic, medications to control the problem must be used indefinitely. As a child gets older, the hyperactive component of ADHD becomes less severe, so medication can be reduced somewhat or used as needed, such as when the person is trying to concentrate during an important business meeting. Psychological counselors earn huge incomes teaching families how to cope with the AD(H)D child, and special tutors focus much attention on creating an atmosphere within which the afflicted child can learn.

These efforts may be important but only insofar as they provide a bridge to a time when the child is able to function without these special aids. Even in neurotherapy, children often take medication during early phases of treatment. Also, these children often strongly benefit from tutoring with a special focus on learning how to learn. Finally, families often profit from family counseling with special emphasis on parenting-skills training in conjunction with the neurotherapy. The child then returns to acting normally in the classroom, without any of the special or stigmatizing treatments that have negative consequences for the development of a healthy self-esteem.

### Is It ADHD at All?

Other psychological and physiological conditions can mimic ADHD behaviors. For example, psychometric indicators of attention difficulties are sensitive to anxiety effects. It is often difficult if not impossible to determine the underlying causes of such test results. Some children are anxious and frightened because they are being bullied at school. Children have been severely injured by bullying, and quite often the parents are not aware of the problem. Bullies may threaten the child with harm if they tell their parents or a school official. Some parents may inadvertently contribute to the child's fear by responding with orders to "stand up for yourself."

Many children experience some degree of bullying. Frederick Zimmerman and Dimitri Christakis and their associates at the University of Washington report that 13 percent of the children in the group they studied were bullies.[1] Philip Rodkin and Ernest Hodges of St. John's University found that parents do not have an accurate assessment of the extent of bullying.[2] Teachers too underestimate the prevalence of bullying and intervene in only about one-third of the incidents brought to their attention.

Another factor may lead parents to underestimate the negative impact of bullying. Bullying may not be physically aggressive or verbally abusive but can be indirect, such as damaging a child's peer network or outright social exclusion. Dorothy Espelage from the University of Illinois and Susan Swearer from the University of Nebraska point out that direct physical bullying is more typical of boys, whereas interpersonal and social/relational bullying is more typical of girls.[3] Children with low self-worth, those lacking in social skills, and those who are physically weak are common targets.

Of particular interest from the Zimmerman-Christakis research is that the more TV watched by four-year-olds, the more likely they are to become bullies. Early TV watching increases the risk of developing ADHD, bullying behaviors, poor school performance, and obesity. The American Academy of Pediatrics recommends that TV be strictly controlled for content and viewing time. The Academy recommends that children under the age of two watch no TV at all and that older children's TV time be limited. The Academy further recommends that TV watching be a family activity and that children not have TVs in their bedrooms.[4]

**FREQUENTLY ASKED QUESTION**

Q: My son has been diagnosed with ADHD. He doesn't seem to daydream excessively or not pay attention, but he just lies around and is not interested in anything. Ritalin doesn't seem to help at all. What can I do?
A: The problem sounds more like depression than ADHD. A brain assessment would help isolate the cause, which might then be corrected with neurotherapy. Being bullied by his peers is also a possible cause.

Another common cause of anxiety is a child's peer group, which can be cruel in judging physical appearance, clothes, and skill level in games. Children may be severely depressed or humiliated because they cannot find peer acceptance. Furthermore, family dysfunction is frequently a cause of anxiety. Although children in these situations may find it difficult to perform satisfactorily in school, the cause is not ADHD. Rather, the scholastic problems are psychosocial in nature. One can treat these children as ADHD kids for years without noticeable benefit.

Other conditions that mimic the behaviors associated with ADHD include head injuries, thyroid dysfunction, low iron, physiologically based depression, personality disorders, abandonment syndrome, and attachment disorders. The following characteristics associated with a mild brain injury are taken from documents written by several associations that provide support and referral services for head-injured persons, many of whom have been misdiagnosed. Some of these characteristics are similar to those of ADHD.

Chronic fatigue

Sleep dysfunctions

Lack of stamina

Problems planning, organizing, and initiating tasks

Difficulties with multi-tasking and sequencing—i.e., keeping track of more than one thing at a time

Need for structure and direction to accomplish tasks

Poor concentration, attention, and memory

Problems retrieving information from memory

Slowness in processing information, particularly new information

Problems with pacing activities

Difficulty with judgment and decision making

Perseveration—i.e., the mind gets stuck on one issue

Distractibility, confusion

Irritability

Impulsivity

Difficulty dealing with change

Inability to interpret social cues, leading to socially inappropriate behavior

Self-isolation because of feeling different and therefore being treated differently

Difficulty "keeping up" in social situations

Poor coping strategies, which affect interpersonal and vocational efforts

Vertigo (dizziness), light-headed feeling

Tinnitus (ringing in the ears)

Light or sound sensitivity

Smell and taste alterations

Visual, speech, and hearing disturbances

Stress-related disorders: depression, frustration

Emotional volatility—e.g., crying for no apparent reason

Emotional/behavioral outbursts

Compulsive talkativeness

Balance and motor-coordination problems

Personality change

Chronic pain, including headache

Inability to return to work or working at reduced capacity and with great effort

Family breakdown

Possible misdiagnosis as, for example, psychiatric illness or malingering

You would think that people who have suffered a mild brain injury would be aware that it is causing some of their problems. However, neurotherapists find that many people do not make the connection between brain trauma and a change in behavior. Further, some legacies of trauma—such as poor sleep, lack of interest and motivation, problems with mood, inability to organize activities and sustain attention—are commonly considered to be purely psychological in nature. As adults, these people are often considered to be malingerers, particularly if litigation, insurance claims, or social-assistance programs are involved. Children who have sustained a blow to the head can likewise display characteristics that appear to be ADHD. Yet regular treatments focused on ADHD for children with brain trauma are largely ineffective. Worse, some treatments can exacerbate the conditions they are designed to treat. The use of antidepressants with such patients, for example, can negatively affect sleep, interest, memory, and ability to sustain attention.

Patients with symptoms associated with PTSD also show learning and attention deficiencies. These deficiencies can be both psychological and psychoneurological in nature. A psychological effect of trauma may be heightened anxiety resulting in the inability to sustain focus, being easily distracted, sleep deprivation, and fatigue, all of which can affect the ability to concentrate and comprehend. Trauma that results in psychoneurological deficiencies is associated with deficiency in the alpha response, as noted previously. Traumatized individuals often show blunted or negative alpha responses, which result in compromised visual memory and visual processing of information. Both these results of trauma can adversely affect learning and attention and thereby mimic ADHD. Again, treating these individuals as typical ADHD clients is largely ineffective.

Other conditions that mimic ADHD are associated with severely compromised emotional security and self-esteem. Any clinic that focuses on learning and attention disorders sees a disproportionate number of adopted children. Some psychological hypotheses have been offered to explain why adopted children have these problems. They are generally based on the effects of abandonment. If a child learns, or knows, that he has been "given away" by his biological parents, inevitably feelings of abandonment rise to the surface. Further, many mental health care providers have come to believe that this process can begin in utero and certainly at birth, even though the child presumably has no "conscious" memory of attachment to his biological mother. This process results in severely compromised feelings of psychological security, integrity, self-worth, and the ability to be loved. These persistent problems, in turn, negatively affect peer relationships, family relationships, and emotional self-regard. *Self-loathing* is not too strong a term for the deep-seated belief some of these individuals have. This emotional crippling is often reflected in poor social skills, inability to cooperate, a desperate need for attention and recognition, a chronic need for emotional distraction, and a marked lack of organizational skills and ability to sustain attention.

However, adopted children may genuinely have ADHD. One possible reason is that AD(H)D has a significant genetic component. As the theory goes, the biological parents of the adopted child tend, on average, to be learning disabled or attention disordered themselves, as evidenced by their inability to take responsibility for the child subsequently placed for adoption, and they pass on this disposition to their children. Considerable evidence indicates that ADHD can have an inherited component. Joseph Biederman and his associates at the Massachusetts General Hospital studied ADHD in families. They found that 25 percent of first-degree relatives of an ADHD male child had ADHD compared with about 5 percent in families without ADHD children. This hereditability factor is found somewhat less with girls than with boys.[5] This level of 25 percent was also reported by Robert Hunt.[6] Hunt points out that the heritability differs somewhat depending on the type of ADHD and that a family history of mood disorders or alcoholism is an increased risk factor for children. Florence Levy, in a study of twins conducted in Australia, found that the concordance of ADHD for identical twins was 82 percent and for fraternal twins it was 38 percent, again indicating significant heritability.[7] Another hypothesis is that children placed for adoption are more likely than nonadopted children to have been gestated under poor nutritional conditions. The biological mothers, according to this thesis, are likely to use substances detrimental to the fetus or to be inattentive to their own nutritional needs, thereby negatively affecting fetal development. Many of the authors cited above in this paragraph also point out that prenatal exposure to alcohol and nicotine and early postnatal exposure to heavy metals or head trauma increase the risk of developing ADHD.

Other psychosocial problems besides feelings of abandonment in adopted children can give rise to the deep-seated negative self-regard that has consequences that mimic ADHD. Children with a mentally disturbed parent, those from broken and dysfunctional families, those from families living in poverty, and those with an alcoholic parent can suffer from attachment problems, abandonment disorder, or other conditions that result in self-loathing. Some of these children (and adults) can also be compulsive achievers. Their feelings of being loved, recognized, and valued are completely dependent on their accomplishments. Failure or less than remarkable performance can be so terrifying to these children that they abandon all other activities to sustain school achievement.

Personality disorders that mimic ADHD are more likely to occur with adults or adolescents than with children. These disorders are also the product of profound negative core beliefs about the self, possibly with a genetic predisposition. Disorders such as narcissistic or histrionic personality disorder reflect different defence mechanisms a person may use to cope with the feelings of self-loathing. These individuals gain some relief from their disabling fears by avoiding activities (work cannot be criticized if it is never completed), being hypercritical of others (bolstering one's own self-esteem by cutting down others), and making their own accomplishments seem large. Such behaviors can look like the lack of organization, inability to sustain attention, and hyperactivity (often with verbosity) associated with ADHD. Obviously, the treatment of personality disorders is quite different from the treatment for ADHD, even though some of the characteristics are similar.

Another condition that mimics ADHD is attachment disorder. In *Scattered Minds,* Gabor Maté presents a detailed account of the conditions that contribute to the development of an attachment disorder. Basically, this problem results from deficiencies in emotional bonding between an infant and the parent, most notably the mother. Maté describes his own experience of being an infant during the Nazi regime in Warsaw, Poland, when mass genocide was committed against the Jews throughout Europe. He postulates that the emotional trauma experienced by his mother during that unthinkably horrible period resulted in flawed emotional bonding, reflected later in his having characteristics that mimicked ADHD. He further maintains that problems in family dynamics in other, less horrifying situations can likewise impede parent/child bonding, and the resulting problems mimic ADHD.[8]

Another condition frequently confused with ADHD is clinical depression. Some forms of depression have brainwave profiles that are similar to the profiles for learning disorders. Problems include lack of attention, comprehension, motivation, interest, and organization; fatigue; distractibility; low stress tolerance; and agitation.

Another important condition that mimics ADHD is none other than the impulsive, active, and quasi-focused behavior of normal children. When I treat a child with ADHD, I always make sure that the parent understands that when treatment is successfully completed, the child is not going to behave like an adult. The child will still display age-appropriate behavior, which under the best of circumstances can be trying to parents and teachers. One of the great tragedies of our time is that we have become intolerant of the behavior of young, particularly male, children. In some communities around my clinic, more than 30 percent of male children are medicated. And the female children are not too far behind, at 20 percent. Such intolerance by teachers and parents is not only tragic but an outrage. Some children are active, some less so. Some are musically talented, some are not. The activity of children is normally distributed, with some portion of children needing more stimulation than average. These children may be labeled hyperactive, and yet they are within the normal distribution in the population. As with any other distribution, the extreme—true hyperactivity—is expected to be 2 percent or less. Any community that prescribes drugs for more than that number of children is sedating normal behavior. If we think of our evolutionary history, we can see that there is nothing normal about sitting in school for seven hours every day.

Indeed, the common form of attention deficiency, given the acronym CADD, may well have deep ties to our past as a species. Thom Hartman in his book *Attention Deficit Disorder* has suggested that when we were a hunting and gathering society, the characteristics associated with CADD could be extremely important. If one were hunting (or being hunted by a predator), being easily distracted by environmental stimuli and being capable of hyper-focus had significant survival value.[9] Such characteristics, although useful to the hunter, are not adaptive in schools and many work environments. I often tell children whom I treat that their CADD came from their ancestors, who might have been the great hunters and explorers of their day.

## Diagnosing ADHD

As discussed previously, ADHD takes many forms. Some are common and some quite rare. Some respond rapidly to treatment while others take more time. Some drive teachers and parents crazy while others elicit sympathy and caring. In some cases, the difference between a label of ADD and ADHD is the severity of the disorder. In other cases, the hyperactivity is associated with different areas of the brain than are inattentive forms of ADD. In addition, brain maps, more often than not, show that a child's problems with attention involve a variety of inefficiencies in the brain. Often an inefficiency by itself would not cause the child any serious problems, but, combined with other areas of inefficiency, it can cause serious attention and learning problems. The point is that ADHD is not a disease. It is a cluster of behavioral symptoms that require management through self-regulation, which can be attained through neurotherapy.

Conventional practitioners determine whether a child has ADHD by collecting observational data, self-report questionnaires, symptom checklists, and interview reports from the client, the parents, and, if possible, the child's teachers. These data are then analyzed to determine whether the child's behavior fits the symptoms or characteristics associated with the disorder. For ADHD, if it is determined that the child displays six out of nine characteristics related to inattention or six out of nine characteristics associated with hyperactivity and impulsivity in Table 1, then the diagnosis is deemed valid. If the child satisfies both these criteria, then he is diagnosed ADHD, combined type. If he satisfies only the first, he is diagnosed ADHD, predominantly inattentive type. If he satisfies only the second category of characteristics, then he is diagnosed ADHD, predominantly hyperactive-impulsive type.

A complicating factor here is gender. Patricia Quinn, a physician and director of the National Center for Gender Issues and ADHD, and Sharon Wigal of the University of California at Irvine have presented the results of a survey of teachers. They report that 82 percent of the teachers surveyed believed that ADHD is more prevalent in boys, but 85 percent of the teachers felt that girls with ADHD are likely to go undiagnosed and therefore not receive treatment.[10] Further, Alisa Gutman, from the Department of Psychiatry at Emory University, and John Spollen, from the Department of Psychiatry at the University of Arkansas, have reported that ADHD in children appears to be male dominated, with ratios ranging from four to one up to nine to one. However, they report that in adults the ratio of male to female is about one to one. In my clinic I also find that adult ADHD appears to be balanced between the genders, meaning perhaps that male children are treated whereas female children are far less likely to be diagnosed and treated.[11]

Comorbidity (the presence of other conditions in addition to ADHD) is a major therapeutic and diagnostic problem. The disorders that may mimic or co-present with attentional-hyperactivity symptoms include several forms of depression, ODD, conduct disorders, anxiety disorders, trauma, brain injury, autistic-spectrum disorders, learning disorders, and psychoactive-substance disorders. Lenard Adler and colleagues report data, from the National Comorbidity Study Replication, indicating that 32 percent of ADHD clients also meet criteria for unipolar depression, 21.2 percent meet criteria for bipolar disorder, and 9.5 percent meet criteria for anxiety disorders.[12] Thus, over 60 percent of adult clients with ADHD also meet the criteria for a comorbid mood or anxiety disorder. This percentage is almost identical to another comorbidity statistic: in a sample of parents of children with ADHD, over

60 percent met the criteria for having had or for presently experiencing major depression disorder.[13] As discussed previously, ADHD, like many other disorders, is truly a family disorder.

To use an example, let us assume that the comorbidity is depression. The conventional method for assessing depression is an interview with the client and parents, self-report questionnaires (assuming the child is capable), and subjective questionnaires and checklists completed by the parents. After these data are collected, the judgment is made as to whether the child has depression and, if so, what form of depression she is manifesting. For simple depression, she must manifest at least five out of a list of nine symptoms. Complicating difficulties include gender and age. Depressive symptoms to some extent depend on age, in that children are more likely than adults to show social withdrawal, poor motivation, and sleeping disturbances. Gender is of specific concern because female children with ADHD have been traditionally underdiagnosed and misdiagnosed. The gender bias is reflected in that girls treated for ADHD were almost three times more likely than boys to have been previously treated with antidepressant medication.[14] In short, the bias was toward viewing the girls as depressed rather than as having ADHD.

Hal Elliot from the Department of Psychiatry at Wake Forest University found that sorting out the other conditions that coexist with ADHD in adults can frequently be quite difficult.[15] This sentiment is echoed throughout the professional literature concerning ADHD in both adults and children. This diagnostic process can take weeks if not months. Accurate data can be hard to acquire because teachers are busy, parents and spouses are biased, self-reports are notoriously unreliable, and psychological testing is time-consuming and costly. In addition, as many readers may have experienced, many practitioners do not bother with evaluations but base their diagnoses on brief self-reports or on reports from parents or teachers and then start a process of experimentation with pharmaceuticals—"Take these and call me in two weeks." This process is continued until a useful blend is found or the patient quits.

By contrast, brainwave assessment is simple, accurate, efficient, and cost-effective. To keep the comparison clear, let us assume that the client was a male child who had ADHD and ODD. I did not know this diagnosis when he was brought in, nor did I ask before the assessment was completed. The child, Bruce, was eleven years old. When he entered the room, he seemed angry and sullen. He abruptly pulled away when his father tried to guide him to a seat with a gentle hand on his shoulder. Bruce seated himself and swung the chair around so his back was to me and his father. I glanced at the father. His demeanor was broken, sad, and tired. These thirty seconds of observational data would have led anyone to guess that Bruce had a conduct problem. The brainwave data would not only indicate whether my guess was correct but would show me the other inefficiencies in brain functioning that this unhappy child was enduring. Measurements at the five critical brain areas provided ample data for assessing Bruce's problems. The five measurements provide twenty-seven arithmetic markers of brain functioning.

For Bruce, the critical data are shown in Table 2. Recall that site Cz is directly on top of the head, F4 is the right frontal lobe, and F3 is the left frontal lobe. Bruce showed a theta/beta ratio at Cz of 3.22. That ratio should be below 2.3 for someone his age. An elevated ratio in this region is the indicator of CADD. Generally when the ratio is high at location Cz, we find it elevated in the right and left frontal lobes as well (above the 2.3 range), as in Bruce's case. The second critical indicator is the balance of alpha amplitude in the frontal lobes. The alpha imbalance for Bruce was 59.7 percent, with the right having the greater amplitude. The usual cut-off for clinical significance used by neurotherapists is 15 percent, so Bruce was well above that level.[16] This is the marker for serious inefficiencies in interpersonal functioning, and in someone Bruce's age the usual diagnosis would be ODD. I have focused here on only two of the twenty-seven brain indicators, but the diagnosis was precise, and, more important, I could show Bruce and his father just how we could use neurotherapy to treat the problem.

**TABLE 2: BRUCE'S BRAINWAVE DATA**

| SITE | THETA | ALPHA | BETA | THETA/BETA |
|------|-------|-------|------|------------|
| Cz   | 23.2  | 17.1  | 7.2  | 3.22       |
| F3   | 16.4  | 15.9  | 6.5  | 2.52       |
| F4   | 17.4  | 25.4  | 6.8  | 2.56       |

Note: F4 > F3; alpha = 59.7 percent

The basic forms of brain inefficiencies found in ADHD include excesses of slow-frequency (theta) amplitude over much of the brain, excessive alpha amplitude in the frontal areas of the brain, excessive beta amplitude over much of the brain, inequality of brain activity between the frontal lobes, and deficiency of theta amplitude in the back of the brain. The excessive-theta variety can be simply inattentiveness or can include hyperactivity if the excesses are marked. Excess frontal alpha is associated with problems staying on task, inattentiveness, and hyperactive "socializing" and gabbiness. The excessive-beta variety indicates anxiety and inattentiveness, and the child with deficient theta in the back of the brain is fidgety and cannot quiet the brain. Inequality of frontal-lobe activity can have many different manifestations depending on the nature of the imbalance but can vary from inattentive and depressed to inattentive and oppositional to inattentive and emotionally volatile.

After I completed the assessment and feedback, Bruce's father revealed that Bruce had been diagnosed as ADHD with comorbid OCD after a number of visits with a psychiatrist who suggested treatment with both a stimulant drug and an antipsychotic drug. Fortunately for Bruce, his father refused to have his son treated with drugs. He instead elected to have neurotherapy to correct the neurological basis for Bruce's problems. Bruce had thirty-one sessions spread over thirty months. The treatments were weekly for about half the sessions and then tapered to every two weeks, then once per month. At the conclusion of Bruce's treatment, he was scheduled for an additional two sessions at three-month intervals to be sure the changes in brainwave activity were stable. Many of these sessions focused on helping him to recognize and modify the behavior that was causing him difficulty at home and at school. The neurotherapy sessions corrected the two major brain irregularities, and he is now doing well in school and has joined several sports teams, an activity he really enjoys. Bruce has entered early adolescence, which is causing many of the ordinary parental challenges of that stage of life, but nothing pathological.

## Treating the Major Types of ADHD

Let's review the general features of each of the major types of ADHD and then proceed to some case studies of clients treated in my clinic.

### Common Attention Deficit Disorder

The distinguishing feature of CADD is excessive theta activity over the sensory motor cortex on top of the brain.[17] The case of Bruce described above is an example of this form of ADD. Prominent characteristics of this condition are being easily distracted, daydreaming, and having problems retaining information. At higher theta amplitudes, the child becomes hyperkinetic because of the need for stimulation to reduce the discomfort of excessive underactivity of the brain.

To give an example of how a CADD case is treated, let's look at Molly. She was one of those clients sent from heaven. Children like her make neurotherapists feel that they are really helping people turn around their lives. Molly, who was nine years old, had been adopted by a loving and strongly supportive family. She was polite and shy, a little afraid, as many children are on the first visit, and clearly unhappy about herself. Molly reported that she had trouble paying attention in class and was often reprimanded by the teacher for "daydreaming." Molly had no behavior problems in school or at home, but she found doing her home-work unpleasant, and this trait caused some family friction. Molly tear-fully revealed that she felt that she could not learn as quickly as her classmates and "always" forgot what she had just studied. She felt stupid.

Molly's case is one of the kinds that often go undiagnosed. Polite, cooperative, and often seemingly attentive, children like Molly are dis-missed as nice little girls who have limited academic skills. They are also frequently accused of being lazy and not performing up to their poten-tial. This evaluation usually leads to a serious erosion of self-esteem because the child feels defective. Working hard, she still cannot perform well, so she concludes that she is simply stupid and that her teachers and parents either have not discovered that fact or are trying to be kind by telling her that she is smarter than she knows she is. Either way the child struggles on, performing poorly and becoming increasingly convinced that she is deficient. With poor self-esteem and the feelings of emotional abandonment that adopted children commonly endure, Molly was on a path in life toward disappointment, unfulfilled dreams, and personal dissatisfaction.

The first visit included an assessment of the five hot spots on the brain. From a neurotherapeutic perspective Molly's brain anomalies were relatively trivial. She had excessive theta amplitude over the top of her brain. Her theta/beta ratio was 3.5 when it should have been below about 2.3. Molly's treatment was straightforward. I placed the training electrode at the top of her head and set the protocol to suppress theta and enhance beta amplitude. When the brain was performing correctly, theta decreasing and beta increasing in strength, a balloon icon moved around the computer screen. Molly started racking up points as the balloons moved. As she became capable of effecting the desired brainwave changes, the conditions that needed to be satisfied to move the balloons were made increasingly difficult. In addition, because the initial assessment found that the Alert harmonic reliably reduced the amplitude of the theta waves, Molly used the harmonic at home when she did her homework. Using this treatment not only helped her stay focused and increased retention but also progressively lowered the theta waves and thereby reduced the total number of neurotherapy sessions required. Molly needed twenty sessions, as it turned out.

A year or so after her treatment was completed Molly's parents wrote a letter from which the following paragraph is excerpted: "[We] are both very grateful for all you did for [Molly]. It was a real tribute to you that after only one week of school, Molly brought in her flute to play a 'solo' for her new classmates and she wasn't even nervous about it! Last year at this time that would have been impossible for her." Molly's self-esteem was profoundly changed by the neurotherapy, and her newfound self-confidence helped her to succeed in school. As a colleague of mine has said, "Fix self-esteem and you fix everything."

Molly's case illustrates the simplest form of CADD, which is characterized by a high theta/beta ratio distributed over the central and often the frontal regions of the brain. This form of CADD is the easiest to correct; it takes the fewest sessions and usually responds favorably to home treatment with the Alert harmonic. Molly's theta/beta ratios were of only moderate severity, although the theta excess did cause her considerable academic and emotional distress. At higher levels of theta excess, hyperactivity begins to be observed. The child becomes excessively active in order to stimulate the understimulated brain.

### High-Frontal-Alpha Attention Deficit Disorder
This form of ADHD is marked by heightened alpha activity over the frontal cortex. The typical symptoms associated with this condition are

poor organizational, sequencing, and planning skills and being easily distracted. The child is unable to complete tasks, appears flighty, and, although not having reading problems, has a problem remembering what has been read. A serious form is associated with high alpha amplitudes, which cause the child to talk too much. As one client put it, "I have motor mouth." Many of these children have impulse-control problems. Often engaging and sociable, they just cannot wait to say what is on their mind. This interfering behavior starts a cycle that frequently deteriorates to defiance. High-frontal-alpha forms of attention deficiency are more difficult to treat and require more sessions than the simpler, or common, form of ADD.

Susie had this typical ADHD pattern, which is frequently undiagnosed in girls. Susie was an adult when I saw her. At thirty-six she was depressed and angry. She recalled that in school she was always daydreaming and was routinely disciplined for talking and disturbing other children. She did not feel as though she was a behavior problem except for her inappropriately timed talking and moving around the classroom. Talkativeness, flightiness, and poor organization are common behavioral traits of those with high-frontal-alpha ADHD. Girls with this brain inefficiency are often undiagnosed because such behavior fits our cultural stereotype of females. Furthermore, young girls are generally more verbally fluent than boys their age. I see many more adult women than men with this pattern, but that same inequality does not hold true in children.

The principal treatment of this condition is known as alpha-suppress neurofeedback. Electrodes are placed over the frontal cortex, and the client is taught to suppress alpha waves. A variation on this treatment is to increase alpha waves over the parietal area, or side of the brain. I have found that increasing alpha amplitude there reduces the alpha waves over the frontal cortex. I tend to use this placement when the client also shows a deficit of slow-frequency waves in the back of the brain. However, Susie did not have that deficiency, so the sessions focused on the suppression of alpha amplitude in the frontal regions.

Because Susie was an adult before her attention problem was addressed, she also had a lot of excess psychological baggage. She was made to feel stupid even though she was sure she wasn't. Blaming herself for her failures, she could not understand why she could not get anything done. Her apartment was always a mess, she was always late, she "misplaced everything," and challenging assignments were always fraught with severe anxiety because she knew her proclivity to screw up. Her relationships with men never seemed to last, largely because she felt inadequate; her poor self-concept enabled exploitative relationships in which her male friends were insensitive to her emotional needs. She had dreamed of pursuing a career but was stuck in a poorly paid, boring, and, in her view, dead-end job. She indicated that she had trouble staying on target, being organized, and finishing projects. She feared trying to advance toward her career goals because she "knew" she would fail again. Susie had been treated with a variety of antidepressant and antianxiety medications, but none made a difference because Susie had come to believe that she was a deficient individual. Correcting her neurological patterns was one thing, but addressing the destructive self-concept was quite another matter. Susie's case is an excellent example of a situation in which neurotherapy is not a stand-alone treatment. Susie required psychological help to work through the destructive beliefs she held about herself. On the reverse side, Susie's case is also a prime example of the inadequacy of psychotherapy when the neurological bases for the distress are not addressed.

Susie's therapy included three elements. First, she had a number of neurotherapy sessions in which the excessive alpha power in the front of her brain was reduced. She also had a few sessions in which the slow brainwave activity in the back of the brain was strengthened, and another few to increase the activity of the anterior cingulate gyrus over the front midline of the brain.[18] These neurotherapy sessions corrected the attention problem, enhanced her wilfulness, and increased her stress tolerance. The second element of her treatment, psychotherapy, helped Susie correct the core emotional belief she had about herself. The notion of "out with the old, in with the new" fits here. The old dysfunctional thoughts and emotional feelings she had about being a stupid and hopeless loser were changed to emotional self-acceptance and self-realization of her inherent abilities. Career counseling rounded out the three-tiered therapeutic intervention. Susie worked with a therapist to determine her skills, attributes, and career preferences. A few of these sessions were devoted to developing a plan of action for Susie to move forward in her career path. Because the neurological bases of Susie's problems were remedied, the other aspects of her treatment proceeded quickly. When adults like Susie see that the reason for their condition is largely neurological, the psychological and career-motivational elements of treatment are greatly accelerated. As Susie later remarked, "I did ten years of psychotherapy in ten weeks."

When neurotherapists observe elevated alpha amplitude in the frontal regions, they also check whether excess alpha is found over the entire brain. Diffuse, elevated alpha brainwaves may be an indicator of anxiety rather than, strictly speaking, ADHD. Like frontal elevated alpha, they can interfere with focus and comprehension because anxiety reduces one's ability to be cognitively efficient. Joseph Thomas, a private practitioner in Illinois, described clients with chronic anxiety who had this pattern of high frontal alpha. Thomas's report corrected the popular misconception that alpha-enhancement treatment would universally calm agitated or anxious clients. He rightly observed that such conventional "relaxation" treatment might increase the anxiety of some clients; his observation again emphasizes the point that in neurotherapy one size definitely does not fit all.[19] Often, elevated alpha is not pronounced in the frontal areas with anxiety clients, so even if the most salient diagnosis is high-frontal-alpha ADHD, it is essential to take into account the alpha levels in other regions of the brain.

### Occipital Theta Deficiency

You may recall the discussion about the prevalence of alcoholism and criminal deviance among those with ADHD. Indeed, a large percentage of adults with untreated ADHD develop alcoholism, and a disproportionate number of incarcerated offenders have ADHD.[20] This complex relationship of addiction and criminality to ADHD has both neurophysiological and social causes. Assume for a moment that a young adult male, let's call him Michael, has a moderately severe form of CADD. Michael has most likely been unsuccessful in school, has concluded that he is stupid, has developed deep resentments, and finds that the only way to gain relief from the negative feelings about himself is to be aggressive and antisocial. He might, however, become shy and withdrawn to avoid the feared humiliation of being judged inept and stupid. In either case, escape into alcoholic, addictive, or criminal behavior (or some combination of these) can blunt the pain of self-loathing and social humiliation. To focus for a moment on alcoholism, the link between alcoholism and ADHD is not direct. For some alcoholics the demoralizing effects of the ADHD make escape into an alcoholic haze appealing. This condition feeds on itself as the consequences of alcoholism further erode a person's self-esteem. In addition, chronic alcohol abuse results in significant brain damage and a brain deficiency that creates a physical and psychological dependence.

The data on the relationship of ADHD to substance abuse are striking. Sam Goldstein, from the University of Utah School of Medicine, and other experts in the area of ADHD such as Russell Barkley from the University of Massachusetts and Salvatore Mannuzza from the New York Psychiatric Institute have published extensively on the comorbid antisocial and drug-abuse behavior of adolescents and adults with ADHD. Those diagnosed with ADHD become addicted earlier in life and have a shortened time between abuse and dependence compared with addicts without ADHD. Addicts with ADHD are between two and five times more likely to be arrested, and they lose their driver's license more frequently. Between one-third and one-half of ADHD adults abuse alcohol, and one in five has a history of other drug abuse. Nearly 40 percent of the cocaine and opiate abusers studied meet the criteria for ADHD, and nearly 50 percent of individuals with continuing ADHD symptoms have some substance-abuse disorder.[21] Maria Sullivan and Frances Rudnik-Levin of the Department of Psychiatry at Columbia Medical Center also point out that ADHD individuals with substance-abuse disorders are harder to treat than other addicts because their disruptive behavior interferes with treatment.[22]

These data are striking but one must keep in mind that the numbers can be markedly different depending on how they were collected. If one looks at alcoholics, then the number with ADHD symptoms may be quite large. If one looks at adults with untreated ADHD, then the number of alcoholics in this group is likely to be smaller. If one looks at adults who have received treatment for ADHD, the number of alcoholics may be smaller yet. Likewise, with other comorbid conditions, I find that children with both ADHD and ODD, for example, have poorer prognoses for successful treatment compared with those with ADHD alone.

In neurotherapy, the link between ADHD and substance-abuse disorders is found in a deficiency of slow brainwave amplitudes or an excess of beta amplitude (or both) in the back of the brain. The key measure is the theta/beta ratio. When this ratio is low (well below a value of two), the brain lacks the ability to quiet itself, but alcohol or another drug does temporarily quiet the brain and offers the person some relief. Yet the abuse of alcohol exacerbates the problem because it further depletes the theta waves and thus increases alcohol dependence.

As a form of ADHD, a deficient theta/beta ratio in the back of the brain can be considered a genetic predisposition to addiction. In children, this deficiency is characterized by edginess, poor stress tolerance, marked fidgetiness, racing thoughts, squirming while seated, and often sleep disturbances. These children always seem to be moving, scratching, fidgeting, sniffling, blinking, and are difficult to put to bed. Exhausting the child is often the parents' method for preparing the child for sleep. In a frequently described pattern, the child strongly resists both going to bed and staying there but, once asleep, sleeps soundly. Adults with this deficiency often wake up frequently in the middle of the night and have difficulty returning to sleep.

This condition creates attention problems because the children are hyperactive. Further, they have difficulty staying focused not only because of being uncomfortable when not moving but also because of racing thoughts. The children (or adults) cannot keep their minds focused because of incessantly intruding thoughts. As an analogy, imagine trying to study when you are covered with crawling ants and with six radios all tuned to different stations playing in the background.

**FREQUENTLY ASKED QUESTION**

Q: I have ADD and a sleep problem. Are they related?

A: Of the many forms of ADD and sleep disorders, some share common neurological anomalies. I frequently have clients whom we treat for ADD comment that their sleep has improved. For example, one form of ADD is caused by an excess of alpha brainwaves in the front of the brain. This condition is often also found in clients who have problems staying asleep. They find that they wake after a few hours and cannot easily fall back into sleep. When we treat the ADD by suppressing the excessive alpha, sleep may improve as well.

Craig's father was an alcoholic, and the child had the telltale theta deficiency that is correlated with a predisposition for alcohol or substance abuse. Craig's behavior gave new meaning to the term *fidgety*: his mother said that he "drove his teachers nuts." The teachers wanted Craig sedated, his doctor wanted him sedated, and Mom was being tortured by the conflict between her aversion to her child's taking drugs and the need to keep her sanity. Fortunately, Craig was only eight, and he had a wonderful, sharp brain. For him to sit still must have been comparable to trying to keep one's finger in a candle flame. In such cases we pull out all the stops and assertively increase theta amplitude in the back of the brain. Craig was treated three times per week for three weeks. We were able to markedly increase the theta amplitude rapidly so Craig calmed down quickly. We then treated him once each week for about four months. I subsequently learned that Craig's father and grandfather were alcoholics and likely were the genetic sources of the theta deficiency. In young children, the genetic predisposition to alcoholism often causes severe agitation and restlessness. I still hear from Craig's mother from time to time; he is doing just fine in school.

### Hypoactive Left Frontal Cortex

With adults, an inequality in the frontal lobes, with the left being less active than the right, may be found in association with frequent episodes of depression. This condition can be related to their problems as children with attention and focus; such problems result from the lack of interest and motivation associated with the early predisposition to depression. Children frequently have problems including poor impulse control, lack of motivation, indifference, defiance, and low or flat mood states. There are two causes. The first is mainly neurological in nature; the second is psychological. The left frontal cortex is an important executive site in the brain. Inhibition, rational thinking, and management of communication with other brain locations are all directed by the left frontal cortex. Hence, children with this brain pattern often have impulse-control problems. They may "act without thinking" or, more seriously, have anger-control problems. They may also have problems with writing down or reciting (or both) previously learned information. They are routinely described as disorganized and incapable of following through and completing tasks. When asked to do something, they inevitably get sidetracked unless closely monitored and reminded to return to the assigned task.

A psychological cause is present as well. The relation between underactivity of the left frontal lobe and depression was discovered in the early 1990s by Richard Davidson and his colleagues at the University of Wisconsin. In the book *Brain Asymmetry,* they discuss a number of studies of the emotional significance of such asymmetries.[23] For example, they report that stroke patients with left-frontal-lobe damage are prone to depression. Later work by Peter Rosenfeld of Northwestern University and Elsa and Rufus Baehr replicated the finding that depression is related to a more active right (than left) frontal lobe.[24] Most important, they report that such depression can be treated with neurotherapy focused on restoring balance in the frontal regions of the brain.

Many practitioners feel that when the right frontal cortex is hyperactive, the patient is generating negative emotional thoughts, which are believed to be reflected in increased activity on this side of the brain. The effects of depression give rise to defensive anger, indifference, lack of interest, and defiance in order to mitigate the emotionally painful depressed mood. Depression in a child is often unrecognized by parents and teachers because adults tend to attribute the behaviors to wilful acts by the child. He is not trying, is being defiant, does not care, is lazy, is spoiled, or, worse, is evil or deficient. These are common beliefs held by adults when confronted with a depressed child. Thus, although the depression may be neurological, the response may reflect psychological defences against the depression.

---

**FREQUENTLY ASKED QUESTION**

Q: I never had a problem with depression, but recently I lost my job, and I can't seem to get over feeling hopeless and very sad. My doctor suggested antidepressant medication. Do you agree?

A: The distinction between neurologically based depression and reactive depression is important. It sounds as though you are experiencing reactive depression following the loss of your job. Taking antidepressant medication is a big mistake under these conditions. Depression is a normal reaction; it is the body's way of signaling you to take action to correct the conditions giving rise to your reactive depression. I would suggest working with a therapist or personal coach to plan the steps necessary to get back into the job market. Taking medications will likely just make a bad situation worse. Neurotherapy may help here as well if you have a predisposition to depression. If so, the neurotherapist can correct that neurological predisposition.

### High Right Frontal Alpha

When alpha waves are stronger on the right relative to the left frontal cortex, confrontational and defiant behavior often results. When the difference is greater than 20 percent, the child (or adult) usually has difficulties with inappropriate aggression, defiance, and negativity. Recall the case of Bruce. He had been diagnosed as ADHD and ODD, and his brain map was consistent with that diagnosis. In Bruce's case, the theta/beta ratio on top of the head was high, and the right frontal lobe showed considerably greater alpha activity than the left. Children who only show the disparity in alpha amplitude in the frontal lobes would, strictly speaking, not be considered to have ADD. However, because of the consequences of this alpha disparity, these children generally have major difficulties in school and are frequently diagnosed as ADHD because their aggressive, oppositional behavior is considered indicative of hyperactivity.

The alpha-disparity effect is probably better thought of as combativeness that results in defiant and, in many cases, eventually criminal behavior. As discussed previously, research with prisoners has revealed that many of them have the alpha disparity. Ricardo Weinstein, a private practitioner in San Diego, for example, found that the EEGs of death-row inmates showed definite evidence of brain dysfunction in the frontal regions.[25] Many scientists have reported that underactivity of the right frontal regions of the brain is associated with anger, hostility, and violent behavior. This disparity can be either genetic or the result of TBI. In my experience, this condition is more often found in males, which makes sense because males are more likely than females to have head injuries.

When a child has this disparity, with or without some form of ADHD, it is essential that he receive behavioral treatment in addition to neurotherapy. The older the child, the more difficult he is to treat because of the many behavioral problems that have emerged over time. He usually has problems in school because of defiance and inevitably concludes that he is both stupid and "a bad seed." To protect himself from this painful self-concept, the child engages in bravado and antagonistic behavior. Family problems are inevitable, featuring major hostilities and resentments. Hence, family therapy is also usually required. Treating this condition is an excellent example of the complexity of treating a child with a "learning problem." Only highly trained neurotherapists with significant psychological experience should handle such cases.

### Frontal-Lobe Imbalances and Learning Disorders

Disparities in frontal-cortex arousal are also found in children with learning disabilities. Common problems include various forms of dyslexia, disorders in writing, and problems in processing information. The imbalances are associated with difficulties in the way various brain sites interact. If this activity is compromised, cognitive lags are the result, and the usual rapid and efficient transfer of information from site to site does not occur. The following case describes how neurotherapists might treat a learning disorder associated with imbalances in frontal-lobe activity. In addition to brainwave biofeedback to normalize brainwave activity, the neurotherapist might use tasking procedures, in which the child is performing a task such as reading while the area of the brain responsible for that activity is under treatment. From the perspective of our discussion of ADHD, children facing learning challenges may become disinterested in, or actively avoid, difficult school activities. This avoidance may look like ADHD because the child is inattentive, easily distracted, and disruptive of classroom activities.

Paula was tall for her age but intellectually much younger than her nine years. Although she was outgoing, her behavior was socially inappropriate for her age; she constantly intruded on others' conversations, and she spoke loudly. It was difficult to identify the causes for Paula's developmental lag. Her mother admitted to taking "a lot" of prescription medication during pregnancy. Paula had also had a negative reaction to an inoculation, had extremely high fevers as a result of ear infections, and had fallen on her head as a young child. Paula's brain showed excesses of delta amplitude over much of the brain and also marked excessive coherence between the front and the back of the brain on both sides.

Hence, in Paula's case two different forms of neurotherapy were required. First, we set up the treatment so she could change her delta amplitude with feedback provided by a computer in a game similar to Pac-Man. When the delta amplitude was decreasing, Pac-Man moved across the screen and ate up the dots. For coherence, we set up the treatment so Pac-Man would move when two different areas of the brain were interacting within acceptable limits. Paula loved to play Pac-Man, and she progressed rapidly. Once the problematical brain areas had been normalized, Paula learned appropriate social behaviors. A parent helped her learn new skills for socially appropriate behavior after neurotherapy treatments had corrected the brain inefficiencies.

### Anterior Cingulate Gyrus

The cingulate gyrus lies beneath the upper layers of the cerebral cortex (surface of the brain) and runs from the front (anterior) to the back (posterior) of the brain. The cingulate gyrus is involved in many brain activities, but the anterior portion is most closely related to cognitive-behavioral issues that manifest as disturbances in brainwave signals. The anterior cingulate gyrus is associated with obsessive-compulsive behavior, intellectual openness, and cognitive flexibility. When that section of the brain is hyperactive, the sufferer can show cognitive and behavioral rigidity, stereotypy (fixed attitudes), obsessiveness, compulsiveness, stubbornness, and inability to accept the point of view of others. These conditions are exacerbated by stress. Abnormalities in the structure and function of the anterior cingulate gyrus are also found in some forms of autism and in serious forms of depression.

Usually found with other brain irregularities, a hyperactive anterior cingulate gyrus causes attention problems resulting from stubbornness, cognitive inflexibility, and repetitive thoughts. Learning or paying attention to new material is hard because the children cannot get competing or inconsistent themes out of their mind. These children appear to have behavior problems because their stubbornness seriously interferes with their ability to follow direction and to focus on learning. Parents might feel that the word *stubborn* does not truly capture the child's inability to listen to reason. Difficulty with focus and attention derives from intellectual inflexibility. The children want their own way and are strongly resistant to change.

Rarely do I see a pure form of hyperactive anterior cingulate gyrus, in which children are obsessive-compulsive, perfectionists, and bothered by incessantly repetitive themes. One child complained that she could not concentrate because she would get "songs caught in her head." She also said she "did not feel normal." Some relationship may also exist between marked hyperactivity of the anterior cingulate gyrus and psychotic behavior. Clients who have been diagnosed with a psychotic disorder frequently have brain maps showing marked anomalies in this region of the brain.

The case of Zim illustrates the interaction of a brain deficiency with deficiencies in parenting. Zim was almost seven when his father brought him to see me; he complained that Zim could not read. Zim had hyperactivity of the cingulate gyrus (as indicated by an elevated ratio of the amplitude of

28–40 Hz/16–25 Hz, as described previously) but not much else in the brain that looked problematical. Zim refused to cooperate with his teachers, saying that he did not want to learn how to read. His mother, according to the father, told Zim's teachers that it was all right if Zim chose not to learn to read; he did not have to read if he did not want to. This is simply an abrogation of parental responsibility. To help Zim, we had to fix a lot more than his hot anterior cingulate gyrus. In particular, we had to work with both parents to help them develop skills for consistent and systematic parenting that focused on providing Zim with what he needed rather than on what he wanted.

At the other end of the scale, children with low ratios, indicating low arousal of the anterior cingulate gyrus, tend to exhibit excessive passivity. The clinical profile of the clients with low ratios, in combination with other brain patterns, is at present under investigation. We have found some serious problems of aggression, opposition, and anger management with this condition. For example, behavior in conflict situations can invite exploitation and can lead to increased social conflict and violence.

> **FREQUENTLY ASKED QUESTION**
> Q: I have bipolar depression. Can neurotherapy help?
> A: Typically with bipolar clients, I find problems in the frontal lobes and usually a slow-frequency deficiency in the back of the brain. With multiple problematical areas to be corrected, neurotherapeutic treatment requires many sessions. However, in my experience neurotherapy has been remarkably successful in treating bipolar depression.

The discovery, in my clinic, that we could both measure and treat anomalies in the activity of the cingulate gyrus was exciting. This discovery allows us to treat conditions associated with dysregulation of this subcortical structure. With neurotherapy we are now able to treat such symptoms as mental and behavioral rigidity, inflexibility, compulsivity, and obsessiveness. This work is still new. Thus far in my clinic we have been suppressing these HF brainwaves to treat the obstinate behavior of defiant children, the unrelenting negative focus of some forms of depression, the repetitive behaviors of some autistic children, the excessive fretting of chronic worriers, and the symptoms of OCD.

The words of a client with the high-frontal-alpha form of ADHD express the desperation, anguish, and frustration that children (and adults) endure when they have a severe form of this disorder. Roy's brain map differed slightly from the pure form in that he had a mild deficiency in slow-wave amplitude in the back of the brain. This deficiency caused him to sleep badly. In his account, Roy also refers to his son, who has similar learning challenges. Roy is a successful self-employed businessman despite his challenges.

I have a beautiful wife, and I have three awesome children. I am forty-four years old, and my whole life I had been told by my parents that I had dyslexia of some sort. Then through testing I was told that I wasn't dyslexic. Then all of a sudden I was diagnosed with ADD, but they were not really sure. Of course that was thirty-three, thirty-four years ago. Through Dr. Swingle I have found out that I have definitely had challenges my whole life. In just two days of treatments, which is four different types of treatments, already the way I'm sleeping and feeling is unbelievable. I'm just excited to see what's going to happen in the next handful of months in my life, to be able to move forward. My middle son has the same type of brainwave patterns that I have, and I have noticed that he has the same types of learning challenges that I had when I was growing up. The biggest challenges I had when I was growing up were learning how to read and paying attention in class. It embarrassed me unbelievably. My whole life, if somebody would ask me to read out loud, I would just get fear. My whole body would get hot, and I would start shaking. I'm on four different corporate boards right now, and it is just amazing [that] when I go to these meetings I think about it before I go. During the meeting, if they ask me to read or to repeat something that I said or they said, my fear of forgetting or my fear of not being able to read right or not be able to comprehend what I just read is such a huge fear I almost get nauseated.

This fear has been with me my whole life, ever since I can remember, ever since the first grade until now. It's unbelievable; this fear has been with me in every single grade. I flunked first grade. They held me back in the first grade because I wasn't able

to read, and later I just wasn't able to remember what I was reading. I was very emotional about these types of things. I had to fake
my [way] through school my whole life. I tell most people today
that what I do is copy. I became a professional copier and that kind
of caught up with me in high school in my senior year. I had a lot
of aides help me out through a lot of my courses just because of
the challenges that I faced. When I was growing up they would
take me to a doctor for testing and they would have tutors for me,
at different stages, because they thought I was very slow. My parents were very sensitive about how I felt and were always worried
about scarring me. I was scarred very badly, even though my parents were very sensitive about that and loved me very, very much.
I knew that I was slower; I had to go to a tutor, take tests at the
doctor's office; and I knew that my other brothers didn't have to
do that. I knew that something was wrong. It is amazing that being
held back in first grade, having tutors, being tested has absolutely
scarred me for life. I thought that I was dumb and not as sharp as
everybody else. Everything that I did in my whole life, even if it
was just getting in a conversation with a few people and they were
talking about something that I didn't know about, [led me] immediately [to think] . . . , "Oh, I'm just dumb that's why I don't
know that." I've been fortunate to do very well in my life and had
incredible parents and an older brother that believed in me and
helped me through a lot of different things.

To this day, I can't stand to read. I hate reading because I have
scars [from] not being able to comprehend. In the classroom, the
teacher would say I want you all to read from page 52 to 65, and
I would sit there in horror with sweat coming down from my
forehead. And then the teacher would ask, "What did you read,
what did you get out of that?" I couldn't remember a doggone
thing that I read, and I didn't even get it all done. I was embarrassed that I took two or three times longer to read it than any-
body else, and yet I just couldn't comprehend it and couldn't
remember what I had just read.

Roy goes on to describe specific experiences with tutors, special
education classes, and the like. He also mentions a phenomenon that

I frequently encounter: he expressed considerable relief when I showed him the areas of inefficiency in his brain and described to him, with "amazing" accuracy, the kinds of learning challenges that he had as a child and that he continues to experience. Most important to Roy, however, was discovering that one of his sons had a similar brain pattern, which was consistent with the learning problems the child was experiencing. The potential for neurotherapy to correct these inefficiencies and spare his child from the nauseating humiliation he had endured as a child was "very exciting so that [my children] don't have to be scarred, they don't have to go through the challenges I went through, and they are able to be the best they possibly can."

My work over the course of more than twenty years with thousands of children with learning and attention difficulties has led me to several conclusions. The most critical is that few children have difficulties that can be truly called a "disorder." Healthy children are active, noisy, distractible, rambunctious, stubborn, impulsive, nosey, and emotionally needy. They need good parents, good schools, good teachers, good spiritual role models, and a safe environment. They don't need drugs—prescription or otherwise.

The child with neurological inefficiencies that make learning and attention problematical can be dramatically helped without drugs by normalizing brain functioning. As we have seen in this chapter, the power of neurotherapy resides in its precision in locating the brain regions associated with the child's challenges. The simplest form of ADHD to fix is that associated with elevated theta in the middle and front of the brain. A far more difficult form is the type associated with excess alpha amplitude in the frontal regions of the brain. Plus, ADHD can be only one of several problems confronting clients. They may have a deficiency in the back of the brain and high frontal alpha, as was the case with Roy. Sometimes the ADHD component is the least of the clients' concerns when they come in for treatment. The next chapter examines the broad reach of neurotherapy for the treatment of a wide variety of disorders, some of which also involve problems with attention, learning, and memory. Because many types of clients are discussed in the next chapter, it may address concerns you have for yourself or a loved one. Here too you may recognize symptoms in the cases I discuss. If so, perhaps neurotherapy holds answers to questions you have had for a long time.

CHAPTER 6

# The Broad Reach of Neurotherapy

Neurotherapy has a broad reach. It is evolving into a primary-care alternative to prescription drugs for many disorders. Rather than sedating overactive children or forgetful seniors, neurotherapy changes the neurophysiological bases of the problem. When administered by licensed and well-trained professionals, neurotherapy has no adverse side effects. Successfully treated clients do not have to depend on a drug to get by in life. Neurotherapy is a primary treatment option rather than the last resort of patients who are casualties of drug-oriented treatments.

As described previously, attention deficiencies in children and anxiety disorders in adults are easily improved with neurotherapy. More challenging conditions, such as the severe depressions, psychoses, personality disorders, the aftermath of severe mental trauma, brain dysfunctions, and seizure disorders are now also being treated with neurotherapy as a first choice. Neurotherapy is emerging as an initial choice because it works without adverse side effects, the changes are permanent, and clients are not harmed by, nor do they become dependent on, drugs.

In the previous chapter, I presented a portrait of ADHD and its various forms, their associated brainwave patterns, and the power of neurotherapy to alleviate the manifestations of these conditions. In this chapter, I look at the brainwave patterns associated with various forms of depression, traumatic injury, autistic disorders, and the addictions. Here too we discover that neurotherapy is a powerful option for treating these serious, life-altering disorders.

## Depression and Bipolar Disorder

Neurological patterns associated with depression are inequality of frontal-lobe activity, deficiency of slow-wave activity (theta) or excessive fast-wave activity (beta) in the occipital (back) region of the brain, and deficiency in 13–15 Hz activity (SMR) over the sensory motor cortex. Whether these conditions are labeled monopolar depression, bipolar depression, reactive depression, indigenous depression, manic depression, agitated depression, ADD, and so on is largely irrelevant. Depression can take many forms. When a therapist sees a brain map with a deficiency in slow-wave activity in the back of the brain and with the right frontal lobe about 30 percent more aroused than the left frontal lobe, then she can say with remarkable accuracy that the client experiences anxiety with despondent mood states.

In general terms, when the brain map shows one of the several patterns associated with depression, the neurotherapist probes the client to determine whether he admits to characteristics of depression. Clients may not recognize that their behavior reflects clinical depression. Such experiences as lack of interest, a limited number of joyful episodes, fatigue, sleep disturbance, low appetites (whether for food, sex, or intellectual or emotional stimulation), poor motivation, lack of future orientation, pessimism, and low self-regard can all be manifestations of depression. Children with depression-related brain patterns are particularly prone to being misdiagnosed. At our clinic we frequently see that such children have been diagnosed as ADHD or ODD. Further, because of the child's lack of motivation, energy, and interest, parents are likely to see the child as sullen, lazy, unmotivated, or obstinate.

Norman was just such a child. He was dragged into my office by an irate father who angrily accused him of being a lazy, ungrateful, and disrespectful child who needed "discipline not brain cuddling." I liked the phrase "brain cuddling," so I asked the father why he had brought Norman to see me if he thought Norman did not need treatment. The father said he was "forced" to do so by the child's mother, who had said that she would not allow Norman to "try" any more drugs. Norman had been taking Ritalin for a while, and for some unexplained reason he had been on the antipsychotic medication risperidone. Among other adverse effects, Ritalin may increase the risk for depression.

William Carlezon and his colleagues at McLean Hospital in Belmont, Massachusetts, reported that rats given Ritalin showed behaviors resembling depression.[1]

Norman was also quite overweight. Sarah Shea and colleagues from the Department of Pediatrics at Dalhousie Medical School have documented that although risperidone can reduce behavior problems with pervasive developmental disorders, a serious side effect is rapid weight gain.[2] Norman admitted that he often spent his day in front of the TV or playing video games. He rarely went out, he saw friends infrequently, and he played sports only at school during gym period. He never, according to his self-report, played games with the other children during recess or after school. His response to my inquiries about his interests, career goals, and what he did for fun was a shrug of the shoulders and usually "I don't know." Norman's brain assessment showed a marked imbalance in the arousal between the frontal lobes, with the right showing 32.3 percent greater beta amplitude than the left.

Neurotherapy treatment for this condition is quite straightforward. The sessions decrease the frontal-lobe inequality; they are augmented by therapy to assist the client to readjust thought and behavioral patterns that may be sustaining the depression. Norman's father had a remarkable change in attitude once he saw the brain map and understood that the drugs likely had exacerbated the problem. Norman's mother never came to the sessions with Norman, so I suspect some unhealthy family dynamics. Nonetheless, Norman progressed rapidly, although at first grudgingly because of my recommendations for severely restricted TV and video-game time. In addition, Norman became engaged in some after-school activities and was enrolled in a summer activities program. Although Norman was often grumpy with me because I restricted his video-game playing, he proudly announced to me that he had signed up for a baseball team. He discovered that he was a good pitcher. His father seemed quite proud of Norman's baseball skill and reported that he felt that his son was now "just a regular kid."

When suffering from manic depression or bipolar depression, a person is predisposed to fluctuating mood states—either deep depression or poorly controlled manic periods. Clients differ in the frequency of the mood shifts and the duration of a particular mood. Some clients report persistent depression with only occasional brief and moderate manic periods. Others report marked fluctuations with long and intense highs and lows. The lows can be severe states of suicidal depression in which the client requires hospitalization. The highs can be experienced as sleepless episodes of extraordinary, and frequently undisciplined, energy that can be associated with financially ruinous spending sprees, starting major projects such as the total renovation of one's home, multiday nonstop driving trips, or insatiable pursuit of appetites. The brainwave pattern often associated with bipolar disorder is a disparity between frontal lobes in combination with one or more of the following: a deficiency of theta waves in the back of the brain; a deficiency of the SMR (13–15 Hz) over the sensory motor cortex (Cz); excessive alpha activity in the frontal areas of the brain; and excessive beta waves in the back of the brain.

Treatment of bipolar disorder is intricate, in that the therapist must be extraordinarily careful that the treatment of one state (depression) does not precipitate the opposing state (mania). The neurotherapist must always include behavior therapy focused particularly on the mania part of the disorder. When it is occurring, mania usually "feels very good," so behavioral controls to temper these excesses are necessary. As a simple example, if mania results in spending sprees, then all means for obtaining credit (such as access to bank accounts, friends, credit and charge cards, daily income allowances, store credit) should be in some way blocked. Thus, when a major episode occurs during treatment, the serious effects of the episode are minimized.

Peter Whybrow from the Department of Psychiatry at the UCLA School of Medicine reminds us in his two books, *American Mania* and *A Mood Apart,* that depression and mania also have some positive features. Depression signals that something is not right and that corrective action is required. Medicating inappropriately or too early can mask this function. Bipolar states, Whybrow contends, may stem from genes that code for extra activity and optimism. If a person has a few of the many genes that contribute to the illness manifestation, he has positive temperament and drive and survives on little sleep. If he has too many of these genes, he has serious emotional problems. Without some of the "manic genes" in the human pool, we might still be "wandering around munching on roots."[3]

**FREQUENTLY ASKED QUESTION**

Q: My antidepressant medication really works for me. Why should I stop?

A: You should stop for the same reasons alcoholics should stop burying their feelings in booze. Long-term drug effects are problematical; you will likely need more to get the same relief; and it's nice for your family to talk to you instead of to your drug. When needed, antidepressant medications can provide a window of opportunity for a person to address the conditions causing the depression. These conditions may be social (feeling stuck in a dead-end situation) or neurological (a brain-wave predisposition). Once the causes of the depression are resolved or remedied, the medications are slowly eliminated.

All emotional states have some potentially positive properties. Only when they are too long or too strong or when they occur at the wrong time does the system become inefficient and maladaptive. Medicating an emotion because it is uncomfortable creates a growing problem because the emotional states are not dealt with and the cognitive and environmental conditions associated with those states are not modified. Neurotherapy normalizes brain functioning, leaving the adaptive features of all emotional states in place. Neurotherapy does not sedate or eradicate emotional states.

A form of depression that can appear similar to manic depression is actually a reaction to severe agitation of the sort suffered by neurologically predisposed alcoholics. This condition might be called "agitated depression"; it is associated with marked deficiency in slow-wave amplitude or an excess of fast waves in the back of the brain (or both). Individuals with this condition experience life as severely stressful, and they are unable to find personal quiet. It appears as though the depressed mood state is defensive or protective. These clients do not seem to respond well to antidepressant medications and often have a history of addiction to benzodiazepines such as Valium. The treatment for this condition involves increasing theta waves or decreasing beta waves (or both) at the back of the brain in conjunction with some psychotherapy.

Depression can also be a reaction to an outside event. If a friend dies, for example, you may become depressed because of the psychological impact. Grief is not clinical depression, but events that involve grief can cause depression. Individuals who do not recover from the grieving period but become clinically depressed may be predisposed to depression. I have had many clients who sought treatment for prolonged depression after a death or a financially ruinous event and who showed the brainwave pattern for depression. Although unimportant for the treatment strategy of balancing the arousal in the two frontal lobes, it is interesting to consider whether the brainwave disparity was the result of the episode or whether the brainwave condition preceded the event.

Determining whether dysfunctional brainwave conditions existed prior to traumatic events such as abuse, threat to life, severe loss, and profound failure might be important in the prevention of psychological disorders. For example, if a person shows frontal-lobe disparity or slow-wave deficiency in the back of the brain, she may be prone to conditions such as severe depression or PTSD. The conditions are, in a sense, latent and emerge in certain experiential situations. Such individuals may be prone to PTSD after an automobile accident, for example, or prone to severe depression after experiencing a loss.

I often see individuals, usually adults, who show one of the brainwave patterns for an attention deficiency who also are depressed. They appear to be depressed because of disappointments that are associated with their learning deficiencies. In such cases, the treatment for depression is the treatment for the particular attention or learning deficiency. As always, particularly with adults, neurotherapy is combined with behavioral and cognitive therapy to eliminate habitual patterns that have developed as a result of the unresolved neurological problem. I might, for example, assist a patient in career-change planning while the brainwave-biofeedback sessions focus on suppressing excessive slow-wave amplitude over the sensory motor cortex (the simplest form of ADD).

On the wall in my office is a beautifully framed quarter. It is not old (1980), and it is worth only twenty-five cents. But to me it has great value. Clients often ask about this curious quarter. Some jokingly suggest that this was the first quarter I ever made as a psychotherapist. One person cited the *Peanuts* cartoon where Lucy sits behind a lemonade stand with the sign "Psychiatric Consultation 5¢." The truth is I often make quarter bets with my clients. For instance, I bet a distressed artist who was hospitalized because of suicidal depression brought on by artist's block that he would paint again. And he did—he paid the quarter when his exhibit opened in Boston.

My framed quarter was won from John, a severely depressed man of forty-two who had developed many aches and pains that prevented him from working. A health professional by training, John had been hospitalized many times; when I first met him, he was a day patient. Patients like John usually have been hospitalized and need a structured program of activities, group therapy, and individual therapy to sustain them in the community. Unfortunately, many of them become "professional patients," whose entire lives are defined by their disorders. They usually have limited social exposure other than with other patients, and their focus is on coping with their disorders to the exclusion of any dreams about the future. A psychiatrist whose treatment of John for six years had sustained him during major suicidal crises referred him to me after hearing about the potential of using neurotherapy with these chronic clients.

In one form of severe depression, the right frontal cortex is markedly more aroused than the left, and John's brain map indicated that this was the case with him. Thus, the frontal cortex was the area where treatment should be focused. To equalize frontal-lobe activity, we suppress theta and enhance beta waves over the left frontal lobe. We also focus some attention on restoring the quality of a patient's sleep by prescribing one of the harmonic sounds that increase slow-wave amplitude at the back of the brain. In addition, a cranial microamperage stimulator can be helpful for restoring sleep because these instruments also increase slow-wave amplitude.

John's self-rated pain and his daily activities were monitored during treatment. He had wanted to go back to work but was convinced he would never be able to do so. The early stages of treatment with clients like John are critical. These clients are disillusioned, and they feel hopeless, useless, and physically unwell. They often have been in therapy for years without much change, and they give up easily. Encouraging John just to get out of bed in the morning was a challenge because he did not see any reason for it and often persuaded himself that he could not get up. John wanted late-afternoon appointments, so I promptly scheduled him for 9 A.M. "Change takes effort, John. This time we get the job done," was a statement I made routinely as he struggled to comply with treatment requirements.

John responded quickly to the cranial stimulator and the neurotherapy directed at balancing the frontal lobes. His enthusiastic response made the other elements of his treatment move rapidly, for he gained motivation to get out of bed and to start to engage in activities. The treatment of John required two years; during the last eight months he was gradually regaining his career. He started volunteering one day a week and then was hired on a part-time basis. Eight months later he was put on full-time. After learning that John was working, the psychiatrist who had treated him for six years said, "My God, I don't believe it. I think I'm going to faint." I eventually won two quarters from John. He gave me the first when he was accepted on a volunteer basis. The second quarter he framed for me when he started working full-time.

---

**FREQUENTLY ASKED QUESTION**

Q: I have heard that when you stop taking antidepressant medications, the problems return. Is this also true of neurotherapy?

A: Once neurotherapy fixes a brainwave anomaly, it's fixed. Relapses are rare provided the brain changes have been stabilized.

---

**Traumatic Brain Injury**

Neurotherapy can be of considerable benefit in the treatment of mild TBI. A full nineteen-site brain map is made for any client with a suspected injury. Initially, the full brain map is analyzed for high theta/beta and delta/beta ratios. An injury sustained in an automobile accident in which the person struck the left frontal area of the head might show, for example, high theta/beta ratios in the left frontal lobe. The blow does not have to be to the front of the head. A "contre-coup" injury stems from a backlash type of movement on the opposite side of the head. In the above example, a blow on the left side of the left frontal lobe could result in contre-coup at locations in the right parietal areas of the brain. Because of the way the brain sits in the cranial vault, an impact from almost any direction causes frontal damage. Because the frontal areas of the brain are the executive areas, the injury results in problems with planning, organization, emotional control, memory, and the like.

Dysfunctions resulting from mild TBI can include excessive slow-frequency amplitude over the areas of damage, excessive fast-frequency amplitude over much of the brain, and deficient interconnections among different areas of the brain. Interconnections, referred to as coherence, can be deficient or excessive. Thus neurotherapy can involve the suppression of the theta/beta ratios at the affected locations. If the brain map indicates that the effects of the TBI include deficiencies of coherence among various areas of the brain, then neurotherapy is focused on normalizing the coherence. By using special electrode placements and working with two sites simultaneously, the neurotherapist can treat these features of intersite brain interactions. Performing this procedure, although simple in purpose, is rather complex in practice. Suffice it to say that we often find people diagnosed with ADHD or clinical depression who, in fact, would be more appropriately considered as having mild TBI or postconcussive syndrome. The treatment of these conditions is often quite different from the treatment of simple attention deficiencies, and again the power of the neurotherapy resides largely in the diagnostic precision afforded by the brain assessment.

Some of the studies on the efficacy of neurotherapeutic treatment of brain injury have been encouraging. Jonathan Walker, a neurologist in private practice in Dallas, and his associates conducted a study of twenty-six patients with TBI treated with neurotherapy. Of these patients, 88 percent reported at least a 50 percent improvement in symptoms, and all the patients who had worked prior to the brain injury returned to work after treatment.[4] Another promising neurotherapeutic technique for the treatment of head injury and, in particular, the immediate treatment of concussion is cerebral-blood-flow feedback. This technique, called hemoencephalography (HEG), measures cerebral blood flow and instantly provides the client with feedback. Hershel Toomim of the Biocomp Research Institute in Los Angeles developed an instrument to provide HEG feedback that has been used successfully with brain-injured clients as well as with children with ADHD and migraine sufferers.[5]

## Autistic Disorders

The incidence of autistic disorders, including Asperger's, has increased since the mid-1990s. Eric Fombonne of McGill University reports that the estimated rate of autism increased about threefold from the 1960s to the 1990s. The Centers for Disease Control and Prevention analyzed data from 2000 to 2002 and found that the incidence rate for autism disorders, including Asperger's and unspecified pervasive developmental disorders, was one in 150 children.[6] As with ADHD, children's levels of autism can vary considerably based on social awareness, intellectual skill, creativity, hyperactivity, impulse control, and sense of humor. Also as with ADHD, the problematic behaviors and areas of development can be detected from the brain map. When treating children with these disorders, therapists look for often-subtle indicators of social awareness. These include eye contact, blushing, crying, or other emotional responses to stories, films, or social interactions; unprompted queries about others' feelings, plans, and opinions; and reactions to humor.

**FREQUENTLY ASKED QUESTION**

Q: What is the difference between autism and Asperger's?

A: Both these conditions vary in symptoms and severity, so there can be some degree of overlap. However, one feature that often distinguishes the two conditions is that of interpersonal behavior. The autistic child has limited awareness of others, while the Asperger's child has more interest in interacting with others.

Several different brainwave patterns commonly characterize children with a diagnosis of autism. The following three cases represent a sample of the various EEG patterns encountered with these children.

### Nancy

A breakthrough in the treatment of many autistic children is indicated when I get a hug. When I do, I can bet the farm that the child will experience considerable improvement from the neurotherapeutic treatment. Nancy was eleven years old when I first assessed her or at least tried to do a brain assessment. During the fifty-minute session, there was not a single item in my office that Nancy did not touch, move, hit, or throw despite her mother's heroic efforts to quiet the child. I mention this behavior because these children and their parents are often gruffly treated by health professionals who become intolerant of autistic-like behaviors. Firmly correcting the child in a gentle and genuinely caring manner is the critical first step in neurotherapy.

Nancy's brain map showed a combination of affected areas. She was deficient in slow-wave amplitude in the back of the brain and had excessive slow-frequency amplitude in the frontal area of the brain, mostly in the right frontal cortex. In addition, she had marked elevation of activity along the frontal midline, indicating dysfunction in the anterior cingulate gyrus. This combination of anomalies revealed three problems: inability of the brain to quiet itself, lack of the concept of an emotional self, and repetitive behavior and inability to regulate emotions. As we have seen, deficiency of theta waves or an excess of beta waves in the back of the brain is associated with poor stress tolerance, edginess, sleep disturbances, and general inability to calm down. The depressed activity of the right frontal cortex is also commonly found in children with autistic behaviors. Stanley Klein and John Kilstrom have reported that the concept of self and others as independent emotional beings resides in the right frontal cortex.[7] Finally, the anterior cingulate gyrus plays a strong role in the interaction among thoughts, motor behavior, and emotional states. This structure, when hyperactive, for example, is associated with the repetitive behavior of many autistic children and becomes increasingly severe when the child is emotionally distressed. Nancy's behavior was predictable from the patterns of her brain anomalies. She was always in a frenetic state of movement, did not react to the feelings of others, and compulsively acted the same way over and over.

Treating Nancy's condition was complicated. The excessive theta amplitude over the frontal brain areas and over the sensory motor cortex had to be suppressed without further depleting the theta waves in the back of the brain. The hyperactivity of the anterior cingulate gyrus had to be reduced without further suppressing activity of the frontal cortex. Conversely, the frontal areas had to be aroused without increasing the problematical activity of the cingulate gyrus.

Nancy has had thirty-eight sessions to date and is, at the present time, treated once per month to sustain the considerable gains she has made as a result of neurotherapy. I get a hug each visit from Nancy. She has joined a regular class at her school, developed a group of friends, abandoned medications (the worst way to deal with autism), and, once a month, she helps me feed my fish. Nancy's mother believes that her daughter's remarkable progress is not the result of the neurotherapy alone. She strongly feels that such dramatic progress is equally the result of our "gentle, respectful, and caring" treatment of her child, herself, and her family. That compliment makes me feel good, for everyone on my staff has been trained in the power of caring, intention, healthy energy, and empathetic respect.

## Billy

Eight years old, Billy had more diagnostic labels than I have had hot meals: autism, Asperger's, fetal alcohol syndrome, pervasive developmental disorder, ADHD, ODD, to name a few. Billy's history was unclear. He had lived in many foster environments, some of which, as I understood it, were severely abusive. His biological parents were assumed to be serious addicts, but little was known about them. Billy was out of control but, oddly enough, was easily quieted long enough to obtain a good brain map. He responded immediately to caring, gentle touch, and joking. He was completely cooperative in being quiet during brief EEG recording periods and moved only during the "wiggle breaks." It was assumed that Billy's severe hyperactivity was a legacy of fetal exposure to substances such as alcohol, cocaine, and heroin and that he was intellectually compromised, probably for the same reason.

Billy's brain map showed many problematical features. The technical details were daunting, so let me just say that Billy had eight serious problem areas that, when combined, represented major brain inefficiencies. With this amount of brain dysfunction, I knew treatment had to include in-depth behavioral and psychological therapy for Billy and his adoptive family. Billy was not a twenty-session miracle case. Rather, he is an

**FREQUENTLY ASKED QUESTION**

Q: My son is being treated for autism. Recently he is crying more than usual and seems shy around people. His therapist says this is OK. Should I be concerned?

A: When autistic children start to respond to the presence of other people, it is usually a good sign. If your son is verbal, you might try telling some simple jokes to see whether he is developing a sense of humor. If so, that's great news.

example of the growing number of extraordinarily severe cases that are being brought to clinical psychoneurotherapists. We are sometimes the "end-of-the-road treaters," assuming responsibility for desperate clients, many of whom have been victimized by the health system.

Billy's brain map showed a normal anterior cingulate gyrus, and therefore his neurotherapeutic treatment was relatively uncomplicated. We could use aggressive treatment to decrease the large and pervasive excess of slow-frequency brainwave activity without concern about worsening Billy's condition by further activating an already hyperactive anterior cingulate gyrus. This was indeed good news for, with such a grave condition, it is advantageous to be aggressive in treatment. The treatment sequence started with brain brightening, in which brain-driving procedures were used to suppress slow-frequency amplitude over the entire cortex. We started at the top, moved to the back, and then quieted the frontal cortex. Billy's zero alpha response was ignited by doing alpha neurofeedback with the eyes closed to enhance the alpha amplitude at the back and top of the head. The low-peak alpha frequency was increased at several locations.

Fortunately, the Alert harmonic had a major suppressing effect on Billy's slow-frequency waves. His parents exposed the child to the harmonic sound for considerable periods of time at home, whenever possible when Billy was reading, doing homework, listening to stories, or engaging in some other cognitively challenging task. Television and video-game time was severely limited, and the parents introduced family games and storytelling whenever possible.

Billy's theta/beta ratio has been cut in half over the entire cortex. Still under treatment, Billy, according to his parents, is calmer, responds more appropriately to direction than he had in the past, and can sustain focused attention for increasingly long periods. He remains seated at meal times and has taken an interest in playing a board game that his father is letting him win. His teachers and aides, who had not seen Billy for several weeks over a Christmas vacation, were startled at his immense change in behavior. They asked the parents about these changes, and when they learned about the neurotherapy, several teachers and aides visited my clinic to observe the treatments. They subsequently have made many referrals of children diagnosed with autism, including our next case Jerry.

## Jerry

As a mother once said to me, parents seize on any positive feature of their child that they can be proud of. Some parents have used the adjective *high-level* to describe mild forms of autism. Although autistic, the child is functioning effectively at some levels. The term does not define one type of behavior. Some children appear boisterous and nosey, others are completely unresponsive to social interaction, whereas still others appear quite normal but do not display any emotion. High-functioning autistic adults often appear excessively intense and emotionally flat, and their social interactions seem unnatural and contrived.

Jerry was twelve years old when he arrived in my office with a diagnosis of high-level autism. He seemed socially appropriate, a bit hyperactive, and nosey, and he responded to humor. Responsiveness to humor is an important indicator to me. Many autistic children are extremely concrete in thought and simply do not understand jokes. A child's responding to a joke indicates increased social awareness. During the course of treatment I frequently refer to children with a nickname such as Sluggo or tell them, "It is your turn to tell me a joke." When they start to respond to these joking gestures, I know we are making progress. Jerry participated in humorous exchanges and did not, in my opinion, show the typical signs of autism. On further questioning, the parents said that Jerry seemed to "go blank" on occasion for a few moments, during which he was absolutely unresponsive. The parents also indicated that Jerry seemed to fixate on minor issues, such as the order in which bedtime activities took place. He would become upset if his mother put his clothes for the next day out of order. The shirt had to be on top and the socks on the bottom of the pile.

Although I questioned the diagnosis of an autistic disorder, Jerry's brain map did indicate three major areas of dysfunction. First, the theta/beta ratio was high over the entire brain, and the summated amplitude (amplitude of all brainwaves combined) was 60 percent over the normal range. Second, Jerry's alpha response was markedly sluggish. Recall that the alpha response is the increase and then decrease in alpha waves when the eyes close and open. Jerry's alpha peak frequency was also slow at about 9 Hz. Third, the activity of the anterior cingulate gyrus was nearly double the normal range. This hyperactivity was causing Jerry's obsessive-compulsive behavior.

Jerry's blank periods seemed to be absence seizures. An absence seizure is a condition in which the child appears to go blank, stares "through you," does not respond to verbal commands, and appears to be in a hypnotic trance. The seizures may occur frequently but typically are of short duration, a few seconds. The conventional functional and structural brain assessments such as the MRI and the visual EEG usually are negative. In addition to neurotherapy, it is appropriate to refer the child to a neurologist for an opinion on the diagnosis.

The treatment for this disorder is to increase the SMR amplitudes and to decrease the theta waves over the sensory motor cortex. In Jerry's case, treatment also increased the peak frequency of the alpha response. The obsessive-compulsive behavior was treated by suppressing 28–40 Hz amplitude over the top of the head. The elevated total amplitude was treated by suppressing the amplitude of 2–25 Hz activity at several brain locations. Finally, the alpha response was heightened by doing alpha enhancement and suppression alternately between eyes-closed and eyes-open conditions.

Jerry's case is an example of the problems associated with diagnostic labeling. Jerry had a sluggish brain that was not working efficiently. Further, his behavior appeared to be obsessive-compulsive in nature, and he likely experienced absence seizures. None of these conditions necessarily indicate autism. His case is a good example of letting the treatment be guided by what the brain tells us rather than by diagnostic labels. Jerry is now doing fine. His special education teacher feels that I "cured" Jerry's autism.

## Alcohol, Drugs, and Addiction

Every parent fears that her child's life will be ruined through addiction to substances that destroy the quality and meaning of life. Less severe but nonetheless problematical is the use of substances that can cause loss of motivation and interest in accepting challenges. Many parents do not know, or do not want to know, that their child is using a drug. On the flip side, many children do not know that their parents are addicts. The problem of addiction in clinical practice is severe. The list of variations and complications is endless. Alcoholic parents try to keep their children from experimenting with addictive substances. Teenagers addicted to marijuana may have to cope with ADHD. Parents of children being treated with methylphenidate (Ritalin), may be using the child's drug. It is not uncommon for children to sell the Ritalin prescribed for the treatment of their ADHD.

Recreational users rarely admit to the serious negative consequences of drugs. Many, in fact, maintain that the drugs have a positive influence on their creativity and quality of life. They are standing on shaky ground. Even drugs not viewed as dangerous, including alcohol, cannabis, and prescription medications such as benzodiazepine tranquilizers (for example, Valium), may be addictive to many people who have slow-brainwave deficiencies or excessive fast frequency in the back of the brain. Individuals often become addicted because the drugs make them feel better. The drugs, at least temporarily, compensate for the brain deficiency. The addicts are medicating themselves. In such cases, neurotherapy is the only method that holds out promise for changing the underlying neurophysiological condition that is often sustaining the addiction. Other methods, such as substituting a prescription drug for a nonprescription drug, detox with counseling, group therapy, psychotherapy, do not alter the underlying deficiency driving the addiction.

Nevertheless, psychotherapy is a necessary adjunct to neurotherapy in the treatment of genetically predisposed addicts to help them resolve the nonphysical factors. These types of addicts do not go it alone. Usually a social culture develops around substance use. A gang of drinkers at the bar or a "cool" group of teenagers getting high can be powerful social forces for continued drug use. Therapy to help the addict modify the social context of drug use can be important in helping him stay off drugs.

What effects does drug use have on the brain? In many instances the links have been well established.

### Alcohol

Basically alcohol causes slowing of brainwaves, so the frequency of the highest amplitude brain activity decreases. Although initially increased beta power results in vigorous and boisterous behavior, at higher levels of drug ingestion and later on in the intoxication process, the slowing results in depressed activity. At first, particularly with genetically predisposed alcoholics, there is a sudden increase in alpha amplitude. This sudden increase can also occur with other substances such as heroin, morphine, and opiates, and in practice this increase can be a marker that an addict under treatment has recently used the drug. The sudden increase in alpha amplitude has a major reinforcing effect for genetically predisposed addicts. They use alcohol because it temporarily replaces slow-wave deficiencies and results in relief from their agitated state.

Chronic alcoholism worsens the brain condition that drives the alcohol use in the first place; it results in decreased alpha and theta activity. A person who starts drinking to ease the discomfort or fear of social encounters may create a neurological condition that is functionally equivalent to that of the genetically predisposed alcoholic. Severe chronic alcoholism can result in brain activity similar to that seen in epilepsy.

Prenatal alcohol use affects the sleep and body activity of newborns and causes an increase in total brainwave amplitude. In other words, the summated amplitude ($\Sigma$A), which is the total amplitude of the theta, alpha, and beta bands combined, is increased. Increased $\Sigma$A is associated with developmental delays and cognitive/intellectual challenges and is also observed in some autistic disorders.

As all parents know, drinking by children is associated with poor impulse control, compromised judgment, and suppression of inhibitions. The social pressure on children to experiment with alcohol is extraordinary, for North American culture glamorizes alcohol consumption in a manner that encourages intoxication among youth. Parents should be aware that despite laws restricting the sale of alcohol to minors, it is easily available. The three major sources, other than illegal sales, are older friends, the parents' supply, and disreputable delivery services. These services include home delivery often by taxi drivers.

### Cannabis

Clients who arrive for treatment when high on marijuana or hashish are often easily identified because of noticeably high alpha activity over the frontal areas of the brain. Despite all the hype about cannabis being a relatively harmless alternative to alcohol, chronic use damages the brain. The increased alpha activity is probably the mechanism that supplies the relief reported by those in chronic pain. However, repeated use creates a brain condition not dissimilar to high frontal alpha ADHD. This form of ADHD is often associated with excessive repetitive and unfocused speech, poor organizational skills, and markedly compromised ability to complete tasks. The excessive frontal alpha waves appear to become permanent after three years of daily use even if the person remains drug free after that time. Tests also indicate quite clearly that the brain processes information more slowly after chronic use, even if the person becomes drug free. The decreased mental efficiency is associated with the slowing of the peak alpha frequency, one of the indicators of brain efficiency.

In short, chronic use of pot is associated with reduced brain efficiency, talking too much, and an inability to plan and complete tasks. It does induce euphoria, which is attractive and may provide an escape from feelings of incompetence and failure. Later on in the addiction, these feelings are often induced by the incapacitating effects of the drug itself. Prenatal exposure to cannabis results in sleep disturbances and increased theta and decreased beta amplitude in infants by age one.

### Cocaine and Heroin

Clients who arrive high on cocaine or heroin or both (I have treated clients high on a particularly addictive combination of heroin and cocaine called "speed balls") are also easily identified because of their markedly elevated alpha waves. Chronic use of these substances results in increased alpha amplitude and alpha slowing, among other damages to the brain. Alpha slowing is a decrease in the frequency of the highest amplitude, so that the average peak, for example, might be at 9.5 Hz rather that 10 Hz. When high, these addicts show behavior patterns similar to those associated with severe high frontal alpha ADHD. They ramble on with highly repetitive content and are unable to stay on track in a conversation. Brain assessments of psychiatric clients who are heavy drug users have found that the psychiatric conditions are generally worsened by the drug use, particularly for severely depressed clients, as reported by Eric Braverman and Kenneth Blum.[8]

Prenatal exposure to these substances affects the brains of newborns. Mark Scher and his colleagues from the Division of Pediatric Neurology at Rainbow Babies and Children's Hospital in Cleveland reported that infants exposed prenatally to crack cocaine had brainwave anomalies at birth.[9] Some of these effects, still observed at age one, may explain the sleep disturbances of these exposed infants.

Cocaine and heroin, like other psychoactive substances, affect the way the brain talks to itself. Chronic use results in hampered communication between brain locations that persists after the addict is drug free. For parents who are sensitive to the behavioral changes in their children associated with substances like sugar, the fact that alcohol, marijuana, and cocaine can cause brain-functioning problems comes as no surprise. Changes in site-to-site brain connections are also found in newborns who have been prenatally exposed to these substances. According to research, the major risks to normal fetal development come from the pregnant mother's use of nicotine and alcohol, followed by cocaine.[10]

### Benzodiazepines

Although many of these substances are used to self-medicate conditions such as depression, stress intolerance, generalized anxiety, and sleep disturbances, the usual consequence of chronic use is an exacerbation of the very condition being medicated. Not only does chronic alcohol use worsen slow-brainwave deficiencies, but so does chronic use of benzodiazepines, such as Valium. I have treated many clients who claim to suffer from benzodiazepine withdrawal. Many have stopped taking the medication for several years and still they have a major deficiency in slow-wave amplitude in the occipital area of the brain. On websites devoted to benzodiazepine withdrawal, patients report that their anxiety became far more severe on discontinuing the medicine. Pharmaceutical companies maintain that there is no such thing as benzodiazepine dependence and withdrawal and that the deficiencies noted in brain activity are the reason the clients were medicated in the first place. Given what we know of the effects of the chronic use of other drugs, I think it is quite plausible that the medication worsened the neurological condition of many of these clients. I have treated a number of clients who experienced severe reactions of increased anxiety and depression after only limited exposure to benzodiazepines. Often the medications were prescribed for relatively trivial reasons, such as for relaxing a person after an automobile accident. In one case, a young woman was disabled for over a year after a two-week exposure to benzodiazepines. One cannot conclude that the direct cause of her distress was the medication. However, many people have become seriously impaired after brief exposure to mind-altering substances. We can help these people with neurotherapeutic treatment, but the message is clear. Brain-altering substances are potentially dangerous, and use of these substances for recreational, exploratory, or escapist purposes is ill-advised.

### Central-Nervous-System Stimulants

Proper use of central-nervous-system stimulants, such as Ritalin (methylphenidate) and Dexedrine (an amphetamine), as well as common caffeine, can help treat severe ADHD. However, such stimulants are sometimes used in a grossly inappropriate manner. About 50 percent of children with ADHD respond to Ritalin, but less than 25 percent without hyperactivity respond favorably, as reported by Robert Hill and Eduardo Castro in their book *Getting Rid of Ritalin*.[11] Russell Barkley, professor at the University of Massachusetts, writes in his book *Attention Deficit Hyperactivity Disorder* that stimulants are ineffective for 25 percent to 40 percent of ADHD children, and, of those who do respond, a large percentage also respond to placebos.[12] The National Institutes of Health 1998 *Consensus Statement* on the diagnosis and treatment of ADHD pointed out that stimulants may have short-term beneficial effects, but the evidence does not indicate any long-term improvement in reading, athletic, or social skills, or in academic achievement.[13] However, stimulants do quiet some children and improve attending and thereby have a beneficial effect on family life and behavior in the classroom. At best, the stimulants are to be used on a temporary basis. If a child is seriously hyperactive and destructive, using stimulants to calm him may be a viable short-term emergency response until appropriate methods are put in place.

As many as 50 percent of children who have been medicated with central-nervous-system stimulants experience troublesome side effects.[14] Although they are generally considered safe in the short term, extended use of such medications may have serious consequences, including elevated heart rate and systolic blood pressure, tics, slowed growth, appetite loss, weight loss, headaches, and gastrointestinal problems, as well as physical dependence. Up to 10 percent of patients report severe side effects that require discontinuation of the medication.[15] No long-term studies on the effects of these stimulant medications on the brain or the cardiovascular system have been reported.

In his book *Talking Back to Ritalin,* Peter Breggin points out many other serious side effects of the stimulants presently being prescribed for children. These drugs include Ritalin, Dexedrine, Dextrostat, Adderall, Desoxyn, Concerta, and Gradumet. These stimulants can lead to drug-induced behavioral disorders, psychosis, mania, drug abuse, and addiction, and can cause the problems they are supposed to treat—inattention, hyperactivity, and impulsive behavior. Many children become lethargic and depressed and can develop permanent tics, including Tourette's syndrome, with inappropriate medication. These stimulants can retard growth, have been linked to cancer, may cause brain-tissue shrinkage, and may be addictive. The drugs, according to Breggin, suppress creative and spontaneous activity in children, making them more docile and controllable than they otherwise are.[16]

Nora Volkow, a psychiatrist with the Brookhaven National Laboratories, points out that Ritalin is a more potent dopamine transport inhibitor than cocaine. The inhibitors increase dopamine in the brain, which, in turn, has a stimulating and energizing effect. The typical dose of Ritalin for children, Volkow continues, blocks more than 70 percent of the transporters, so the notion that Ritalin and the other similar drugs are weak stimulants is clearly wrong.[17] When the medication is stopped, the neurological condition returns, usually exaggerated on withdrawal, so the medications are, at best, interim aids. In short, stimulants sedate children, and, except in serious cases of hyperactivity, such medications are inappropriate. After a series of neurotherapeutic treatments, the child should be able to function without stimulants.

And I have not even mentioned the illegal traffic in these drugs. In a study, over 23 percent of children on stimulant medication reported being asked to sell, trade, or give to other children their prescription medication.[18] Adolescents and even their parents have been found using the drugs nonmedically by ingesting higher doses to experience a cocaine-like high. In a study at a northeastern university, 16 percent of the students admitted to using stimulant medication nonmedically.[19] Timothy Wilens from the Department of Psychiatry at Harvard Medical School reports that it is primarily patients with a comorbid disorder, in addition to the ADHD, such as a history of substance abuse, conduct disorder, or both, who divert or misuse their stimulant medications. Of patients with a comorbid condition, 22 percent reported misusing their medication (using more than prescribed), and 11 percent reported that they had sold their medications.[20]

The increase in the use of these dangerous drugs is alarming. In addition to a threefold increase in the use of stimulants with two- to four-year-old toddlers from 1991 to 1995,[21] surveys indicate major increases in the use of all psychotropic medications with children.[22] Ninety percent of the world's Ritalin is used in the United States, as reported by Breggin. His summary encapsulates the tragedy: "Our society has institutionalized drug abuse among children. Worse yet, we abuse our children with drugs rather than making the effort to find better ways to meet their needs."[23]

In addition to stimulants, the increase in the use of antidepressants with children has been marked, yet the evidence suggests they are of dubious clinical effectiveness and are certainly risky. "At least five unpublished trials using a placebo control have failed to show an advantage for antidepressants over placebo. Among eight published trials, four found no statistically significant advantage for antidepressants over placebo on any primary outcome measure, and only about a third (17/52) of all published measures show an advantage for drug over placebo. Even the statistically significant improvements are of dubious clinical importance."[24]

### Television and Video Games

Although not as pernicious as alcohol and drugs, the stimulation environment of the child is fundamental to healthy development. Too much television (particularly at young ages) and limited opportunities for imaginative play contribute markedly to the problems of children who end up in neurotherapists' clinics.

I cannot think of a better mechanism for facilitating attention deficiencies in children than watching television for several hours each day. The images change every few seconds, the thematic content is trite, and the child is never challenged to use his imagination. Research evidence suggests that if toddlers watch TV several hours per day, to the exclusion of healthy parent/child interactions, an area of the brain may not develop properly. The right orbitofrontal cortex (ROFC), located in the vicinity of Fp2 (shown in Figure 2, Chapter 2), is critical to the regulation of emotions and the autonomic nervous system. The ROFC is not functional at birth but develops during the first years of life only through interaction with others. These interactions, such as between the infant and the mother, must be balanced both in emotional intensity and in duration. Mothers who are severely detached as a result of trauma, fear, or depression can negatively affect the child's development of this critical regulating system. Using TV to occupy the child to the extent that meaningful emotional interpersonal interaction is severely restricted may also result in inadequate development of this most critical brain system. When the infant or toddler interacts with a person, connections in the brain are formed. This process involves branching and myeliniza- tion of the neuronal fibers and increased dendrite synaptic connections. The brain cleans house every so often in the young child by "washing away" or "pruning" unused brain material. Hence, if it is not used, con- nections in that area of the brain do not develop properly.[25]

Quite apart from the effects of TV on brain function, compelling evi- dence shows that violent TV content (including sports) can increase the likelihood of aggressive antisocial behavior in young children. Experts have long known that the immediate effect of watching violent TV content is a short-term increase in aggressive behavior. However, the longer-term effects of such content have also been established. John Murray reviews much of the research on the effects of TV violence on children's behavior and on their brain functioning. He points out that viewing televised violence can lead to increases in aggressive behavior and attitudes, desensitization to violence, increased fear, and a belief that the world is "mean."[26] The guide- lines of the American Academy of Pediatrics are quite clear—limit TV.[27]

Video games also contain ever-changing images and highly stimulating content. Search-and-destroy games facilitate impulsive, aggressive, and hyperactive states in children. In my experience, boys always describe the games they like in terms that indicate violent content. Here also the evidence is quite clear. Jeanne Funk of the University of Toledo and her associates report that exposure to video-game violence results in reduced empathy and expression of pro-violent attitudes. She suggests that such exposure may emotionally desensitize children.[28] Douglas Gentile and his associates reported that students who played more violent video games were significantly more likely to be involved in physical fights. Also, Gentile notes, the amount of video-game play was negatively cor- related with school performance.[29]

Other aspects of video games are socially and intellectually damaging to children as well. Children in my clinic spend hours each day indoors, lim- iting their behavioral repertoire to machine-guided themes. Parents tell me that their children often get angry when told to turn off the video game or the TV. Astonishingly, parents often report with pride that their child plays hours of video games per day, evidently in the belief that robotic attachment to a computer indicates technological or special eye-hand coordination skills. To develop creative, intellectual, and social skills, one has to practice them and engage in meaningful, stimulating activities. Increased exposure to these games reduces the skill set of the child. Further, sitting down all the time is a physical health risk to the developing child.

A dealer once told me that children who become interested in collecting stamps, coins, or paper money always seem to do well in geography, mathematics, and languages. Of course, you could argue that children skilled in these areas may become interested in collecting. Nonetheless, it does seem reasonable that collecting fossils, minerals, rocks, insects, and the like fosters curiosity about the items. As noted in Chapter 1, in my practice we have a "treasure chest." After each session the child can dig around in the chest and take one item. The chest contains no candy or toys, but instead is filled with rocks, coins, stamps, bills, minerals, fossils, semiprecious gemstones, and cultural items. Aside from the basic reinforcing properties of getting a reward for participation in the session, I am convinced that interest in academics is spurred by obtaining dinosaur bones, shark teeth, petrified wood, stamps, foreign money, crystals, and the like. The child becomes interested in the geographical location of the country the coins or stamps are from, the exchange value of foreign money, the geological calendar for fossils, and so on. In other words, the child's interest in education is stimulated by the reward from the treasure chest. Many children start collections of items that they find interesting. One child won a merit badge in Scouts for a collection of fossils that he had obtained from the treasure chest.

Finally, parents need to assert their authority in guiding the child toward healthy options and limiting destructive options. As I often state to a family group at the first session, "Mothers outrank everybody!" Some decisions are age-appropriate for children to make, and some decisions should be made by parents. When families understand this basic concept, the road to improvement in the children's progress takes a decisive turn for the better.

CHAPTER 7

# The Promise of Neurotherapy in the Future

The field of neurotherapy is developing at an accelerated pace. For diagnosis and assessment, therapists are able to compare the brain functioning of clients to data banks of the brain functioning of many different groups of people. When the brain map of a client is statistically compared with norms obtained from carefully selected people who report no psychophysiological symptoms or disorders, divergent areas of brain functioning are revealed. Additional data banks of specifically defined groups are being developed. Such groups include persons with TBI, adult ADHD, autism, various forms of psychoses, Parkinson's disease, and Alzheimer's. By comparing a brain map to the composite maps of these various groups, the neurotherapist can be increasingly precise in determining when a client's reported symptoms indicate a specific disorder. More important, the data-bank comparisons help tell practitioners how to treat the disorder rather than just how to label it. Compelling evidence shows that brain-system reorganization and remediation of problems can occur quite readily. Studies have shown that changes in blood flow and nerve growth occur during neurotherapy. Damaged areas of the brain can be functionally replaced with healthy areas of the brain. In one form of therapy called restraint therapy, for example, the good arm of a client with brain trauma is restrained, forcing the client to use the compromised arm. New brain areas are engaged as the client gains mobility in the disabled arm. The brain can, and does, recover from injury. And the positive care of the therapist, in combination with

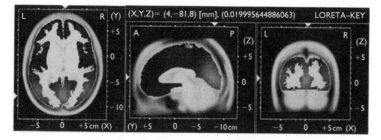

*Figure 6. A LORETA image of internal brain structures.*

an optimistic attitude on the part of the client, has demonstrable and profound effects on healing.

Neurotherapists are developing improved ways to determine the coordination of brain area to brain area as part of the effort to refine the methods for normalizing these brain-site interrelationships. Developments are also occurring in the area of deep brain assessment and treatment. One of these is a brain-mapping procedure called LORETA, which stands for Low Resolution Electromagnetic Tomography. This procedure, developed by Roberto Pascual-Marqui, enables neurotherapists to map the inner cortex of the brain from recordings of brainwave activity on the scalp. [1] Figure 6 is a LORETA image showing internal brain structures. This imaging can be done by a neurotherapist as a simple in-office procedure. The potential therapeutic breakthroughs that this technology offers for the treatment of serious disorders are truly revolutionary.

Although the major focus of this book is the neurotherapeutic treatment of disorders, neurotherapy can be directed at heightening brain efficiency in people without disorders. As I explain to my clients, you can think of neurotherapy as a continuum running from left to right: the left side represents the normalization of brain functioning, and the right side represents the optimizing of brain functioning. Most clients are thrilled when their problems are resolved, and they end treatment at that time. Some, however, continue because they feel that they can progress even further.

Peak performance, or optimal performance, refers to training the brain to respond in a highly efficient manner to challenges. It does not mean that the brain is always on high alert but, rather, that when a coordinated mental event is required, the brain responds to that challenge in the

> **FREQUENTLY ASKED QUESTION**
> Q: Why do some sports teams have psychologists?
> A: Psychologists can really help teams play better. Some psychologists help players keep their minds sharply focused on the game. Neurotherapists also can help by making a player's brain more efficient than it was before neurotherapy.

most efficient manner. The coordinated mental event could be an athletic endeavor, such as shooting a basketball, hitting a baseball, putting a golf ball, shooting an arrow or a hockey puck. Recall my discussion of the World Cup soccer champions, the Italian team, which received neurofeedback training. The mental event could be landing a sophisticated military aircraft. In the area of the arts, neurofeedback training can enhance and optimize the performance of singers and dancers. CEOs of large companies receive optimal-performance neurofeedback training because it facilitates critical decision making in any arena of activity that requires rapid and thorough consideration of complex information.

Peak-performance procedures with CEOs of major companies, professional athletes, and elite military forces train various areas of the brain to efficiently interact with other areas of the brain. One such procedure involves training four areas of the brain to increase coordinated alpha amplitude. Another optimal-performance training procedure is to increase the amplitude of high-frequency activity associated with the integration of information at the point of decision making.

> **FREQUENTLY ASKED QUESTION**
> Q: I received neurotherapy treatment for a severe anxiety condition. I found that my general health seems much improved as well. Is this improvement related to the neurotherapy?
> A: The improvement could be either a direct or an indirect benefit of the treatment. Increasing the speed of alpha frequencies, for example, has been found to be related to improved immune-system functioning.

Many of us have had "ah-ha" and "om" experiences. The ah-ha experience is an instant burst of insight in which an explanation, a problem solution, or the proper course of action suddenly occurs to us. In our culture, the om experience is less common. It is the profound sense of spiritual groundedness, unity, and cosmic understanding that occurs when the mind is uniquely quiet, save for tightly circumscribed areas of activity. This experience is the ultimate goal of many types of meditation. How can it be enhanced by neurotherapy? When a child has CADD, characterized by excessive slow-frequency waves over the top of the brain, the condition is treated by speeding up the brain. By analogy, the child's brain is a digital computer that is running at too slow a speed. The brain is made more active, faster by analogy, so that the tendency to lose focus is reduced. As the ability to focus is honed, the cognitive process kicks in, and the child receives gratification from intellectual activities such as reading and problem solving. By contrast, meditators gain from marked increases in theta amplitude at the back of the brain. This increase in slow-frequency amplitude is associated with mental quieting, during which time the brain rests and restores. Slow-frequency activity in the back areas of the brain is also associated with thinking that is more global, with less attention to detail. Optimal-performance training focuses both on increasing brain efficiency when processing information and on rapid change to the restorative mentally quiet state when sharp focus is not required. Peak performance is the training of the mind to become insulated from distractions while releasing the mind to be in synch with the energy of the universe. The brain is trained to efficiently engage and disengage at the highest level.

The wisdom of om may be acquired in many ways: through the mentoring of elders, through the self-discipline of developing unique talents, and through an appreciation of the spiritual. I believe that it is preferable to acquire optimal-performance skills in the lifelong process of self-disciplined mind quieting, mind-focus training, and learning from wise elders. Our highly contaminated environment, at all levels, strongly interferes with our ability to quiet the mind and luxuriate in the three-pound universe that is our brain. Optimal-performance training is a technological approach to improving a disturbed condition caused by our modern age. It also satisfies our desire to apply technology to optimizing our life experience. It can be of major benefit to all but is of most benefit to those who are open to the profound wisdom available to the quiet mind.

Why should neurotherapy be your first choice for treatment of a wide range of psychological and neurological disorders? I hope that this book will encourage you to ask yourself that question. The simple answer is because neurotherapy (also known as clinical psychoneurophysiology) is an efficient, proven method for correcting the neurological, psychological, and physiological bases for your disorder. Drugs may help you cope, booze may help you hide, and psychotherapy may help you in the long haul, but nothing can compare with neurotherapy for rapidly and safely correcting a problem at the source, your brain. The research of scientists at a wide array of universities has shown that the brain is capable of change. The brain displays considerable plasticity, and neurotherapy harnesses the brain's ability for change to correct the neurological conditions causing your problems.

Everybody knows people who could be poster children for the pharmaceutical companies. Heavily medicated, they limp through life making the rounds of various health care providers. They spend huge amounts on drugs but still are capable of only marginal functioning. An alternative to this tragically diminished life is to permanently correct the neurological basis of the problem from the start. When neurotherapy is the first treatment, a person can become capable of squarely facing life's challenges, as we all must. In addition, neurotherapy is cost effective, its results are lasting, and it has no dangerous side effects. Rather than taking ever increasing amounts of drugs, you will see life through clear lenses. If you keep in touch with your neurotherapist, you can schedule a few visits a year when you are older to brighten your brain to keep yourself mentally and physically healthy.

The evidence speaks for itself. Neurotherapy is a primary-care alternative for the treatment of many disorders that have traditionally been sedated, if they could be corrected at all. It truly satisfies the medical credo *primum non nocere*, "First, do no harm." Problems in brain functioning that cause symptoms can be corrected, with the result that the symptoms go away. Families abandoned with their autistic children can find help; depressed and anxious people can find relief and freedom from drugs; those who have problems with concentration or sleep or anger or alcohol or mental quietude can find these problems resolved. Those with head injuries, stroke, pain, seizure disorders, and age-related declines can also find help.

Neurotherapy is such a rapidly expanding field because its varied methods truly do help people who suffer from neurologically-based ailments. Rather than spending years being shuttled from one health care provider to another, you may want to consider whether the problem you or a loved one suffers from might be helped by one of the methods described in this book. The only shock you are likely to have is the realization that, with a clear head, life offers an abundance of exciting possibilities.

# APPENDIX: PICKING A NEUROTHERAPIST

An old saying among psychotherapists is that clients have difficulty finding a good match because only about 15 percent of therapists are competent, and of that limited number the client will get along with only about 15 percent. This wry observation is overdrawn, of course, but the point is that not all therapists or therapeutic approaches are right for you. This is also true of neurotherapists. Further, brainwave therapy is not a stand-alone therapy but must be integrated with other therapies. In selecting a neurotherapist, you should insist on several basic requirements. These include: an independent license within the practitioner's jurisdiction, certified training in neurotherapy, and considerable relevant experience. If possible, you should also be referred by a former client of the therapist.

Let's take a look at these requirements in order. First, the neurotherapist must hold an independent license within the jurisdiction of the therapist's practice. Thus, the person should hold a license to practice psychology, medicine, or some other relevant health care profession. For example, the person doing neurotherapy might be a neurologist, psychologist, psychiatrist, naturopathic physician, licensed clinical social worker, chiropractor, or general medical doctor. The discipline should be relevant to the disorder that you wish to have treated. For example, a chiropractor would probably not be as suitable as a psychologist for a traumatic stress problem, even though both are experienced neurotherapists. Be sure that the person is licensed, certified, or registered by the governmental jurisdiction where the person practices and not simply certified by some professional organization or nonjurisdictional government. A practitioner who does not hold a license to practice psychology or medicine may represent himself as "nationally certified." This national certification can be a meaningless certification related to a mail-order course. There are several reasons to select a neurotherapist who is an independently licensed health care professional. First, she has something to lose if her treatment is incompetent or unethical. Professional licensing and registration boards or colleges maintain review boards to field client complaints. These professional-practice review boards can censure practioners or suspend or revoke licenses to practice, or they can impose strict requirements and conditions to limit the practice of violators. Unlicensed practitioners have no such government-mandated monitoring agency to which they are responsible. They can be psychological or medical hobbyists whose commitment to your treatment is not grounded in systematic training, proper supervision, and accountability to an agency of authority. The second reason to select licensed practitioners is that they carry professional liability insurance. A psychological or medical hobbyist may carry business insurance, but professional liability (malpractice) insurance is essential for the client.

The second requirement is that the practitioner have relevant therapeutic training to treat the disorder for which you seek help. When you consult with a health care provider, you seek a remedy for a disorder and not necessarily a specific treatment method. If you suffer from migraine headaches, for example, relief from the headaches is the central goal of any therapy. You may wish to pursue biofeedback, but the biofeedback should be administered by a practitioner with other treatment options. Thus, a medical physician may be able to use biofeedback in your treatment, but that is not his only treatment option. Similarly, a psychologist may offer neurotherapy as a treatment possibility, but she has other options such as biofeedback, relaxation therapies, and other psychotherapies and the like to treat the same disorder.

The two agencies that certify training are the Biofeedback Certification Institute of America and the Neurotherapy and Biofeedback Certification Board. Select certificants in neurofeedback or EEG biofeedback. These certified individuals have training and experience at a specific, albeit minimal, level. I would select only a neurotherapist who has been certified by one of these two agencies because such certification demonstrates that the therapist has submitted her or his credentials for scrutiny and that the board has accepted those credentials as satisfying a specific standard of training and experience.

Because of the growing problem of minimally qualified medical/psychological hobbyists purporting to practice neurotherapy, be cautious of franchisees. A growing number of organizations support one-size-fits-all franchise-like operations in which unlicensed, uncertified, and minimally trained individuals use fixed treatments for every condition. These operations do vary in sophistication. Some use only one treatment for every condition, claiming that if brain functioning is temporarily disturbed in treatment, the brain will reorganize toward normative functioning. Other franchisers offer several treatment options that the franchisee selects based on the client's self-report. Thus, if the client claims to suffer from ADHD, the franchisee administers a treatment over the center of the head designed to increase the amplitude of the sensory motor rhythm and decrease the amplitude of theta. This treatment does work for some forms of ADHD but is minimally effective for other forms of attention disorders.

The third factor to consider in the selection of a neurotherapist is the experience the person has with cases similar to yours. It takes five days to train a person to do a few basic neurotherapy protocols. It takes several thousand supervised treatment sessions before one can be considered an expert. Inexperienced therapists tend to rely only on research they read rather than on their experience and accomplishments in their own practice. For example, when children have attention problems, four out of five of them will experience a 50 percent improvement with forty to eighty sessions of theta suppress/beta enhance EEG feedback at the top of the head. When the treatment is done by an expert, a person experienced with hundreds of cases, this statistic can be remarkably different. With common ADD, for example, experienced neurotherapists with fully equipped offices and skills in behavior therapy can claim success rates of over 90 percent.

Some therapists are more effective than other therapists with equivalent or more years of experience. Every discipline, be it music, art, medicine, architecture, psychology, or neurotherapy, has gifted practitioners. Examining the practitioner's credentials gives the client only a basic understanding of how well trained and experienced the practitioner is.

The only way to find the truly talented neurotherapist is to ask former clients of the practitioner. Gifted therapists gain deserved reputations for helping their patients. However, when relying on the recommendation of former clients, keep in mind that a therapist skilled in the treatment of, say, depression may be inexperienced in the treatment of traumatic stress. Hence, even though you hear raving praise of a therapist's treatment, make sure he knows how to deal with your problem.

Occasionally, potential clients ask to speak with clients who have been treated by the practitioner. They believe that way they will obtain a valid indication of the therapist's merit. This method presents two problems. First, therapists are going to refer you to the successes, not the failures. Speaking with a successfully treated client may be reassuring, but it is not a valid substitute for checking the practitioner's qualifications. Second, I am reluctant to put a potential client in touch with my clients because I know little about the potential client. That person could be disruptive to my client's therapy.

The reverse situation is also a problem. I am frequently asked to recommend therapists in other cities. I often know therapists with excellent professional reputations, but I know little about their therapeutic effectiveness. I recommend with the disclaimer that I cannot vouch for them as therapists and that clients must make their own assessments after a few visits. All I can tell the person is that the therapist has the necessary training and credentials and that he or she is recognized in the profession. Clients can often obtain the same information by researching the therapist on the web. The therapist's licensing and certifications, if any, are all accessible to the public. Again, finding truly talented professionals usually happens through previously treated clients.

# NOTES

## Introduction: "It's All in Your Head"

1. J. Robbins, *A Symphony in the Brain* (New York: Grove Press, 2000), 3.
2. F. H. Duffy, "The State of EEG Biofeedback Therapy (EEG Operant Conditioning) in 2000: An Editor's Opinion," *Clinical Electroencephalography* 31 (2000): v.
3. The *National Georgraphic* published, for example, an article on the brain activity of Tibetan monks: J. Shreeve, "The Mind Is What the Brain Does," *National Geographic* (March 2005): 6–31. A. Tothenberger and T. Banaschewski, "Informing the ADHD Debate," *Mind* (Jan. 2005): 50–55; quote on p. 54. Russell Adams, "Getting Your Head in the Game," *Wall Street Journal,* July 29, 2006.
4. W. Wyrwicka and M. B. Sterman, "Instrumental Conditioning of Sensorimotor Cortex EEG Spindles in the Waking Cat," *Physiology and Behavior* 3 (1968): 703–707.
5. M. B. Sterman and L. Friar, "Suppression of Seizures in Epileptics Following Sensorimotor EEG Feedback Training," *Electroencephalography and Clinical Neurophysiology* 33 (1972): 89–95.
6. Elmer Green and his associates published a number of articles on the brainwave state of experienced meditators and on the use of biofeedback as a means to create deep states of relaxation. Many of these studies are summarized in his book, coauthored with his wife, Alyce Green: *Beyond Biofeedback* (Fort Wayne, Ind.: Knoll, 1977).
7. E. G. Peniston and P. J. Kulkosky, "Alpha-Theta Brainwave Training and Beta Endorphin Levels in Alcoholics," *Alcoholism, Clinical and Experimental Research* 13 (1989): 271–279.
8. Duffy, "The State of EEG Biofeedback Therapy," v–viii.
9. V. Monastra, D. M. Monastra, and S. George, "The Effects of Stimulant Therapy, EEG Biofeedback, and Parenting Style on the Primary Symptoms of Attention-Deficit/Hyperacitivy Disorder," *Applied Psychophysiology and Biofeedback* 27, no. 4 (2002): 231–249.
10. Details on the low-energy treatment methods developed by Ochs can be found in S. Larsen, *The Healing Power of Neurofeedback* (Rochester, Vt.: Healing Arts Press, 2006).

11. M. A. Patterson, J. Firth, and R. Gardiner, "Treatment of Drug, Alcohol and Nicotine Addiction by Neuroelectric Therapy: Analysis of Results over 7 Years," *Journal of Bioelecticity* 3 (1984): 193–221.

## Chapter I: The Basics of Biofeedback

1. C. A. Mann, J. F. Lubar, A. W. Zimmerman, B. A. Miller, and R. A. Muenchen, "Quantitative Analysis of EEG in Boys with Attention Deficit Hyperactivity Disorder; Controlled Study with Clinical Implications," *Pediatric Neurology* 8, no. 1 (1992): 30–36.

2. Thomas Collura, developer of many neurotherapy devices, described the effects of repetitive light stimulation on brainwave activity in detail in "Application of Repetitive Visual Stimulation to EEG Neurofeedback Protocols," *Journal of Neurotherapy* 6 (2002): 47–70.

3. Although I often joke with parents that "neurotherapy does not treat adolescence" and that when children's ADHD is corrected, they will remain adolescents, I also discuss the challenges children with ADHD face. Our culture does not provide many suitable outlets for their energy and their needs for exploration and independence. The lure of drugs, misadventure, and oppositional behavior can be strong, and some too fall into depression, which results in lack of interest and motivation. Some may attempt to combat the depression with mind-deadening vidoe games and hours of watching TV. One of the topics covered in the family sessions that often are part of treatment is methods for engaging the adolescent child in vigorous and mentally stimulating activities.

4. V. Monastra, *Parenting the Child with ADHD: 10 Lessons That Medicine Cannot Teach* (Washington, D.C.: American Psychological Association, 2004).

5. J. F. Lubar, and J. O. Lubar, "Neurofeedback Assessment and Treatment for Attention Deficit/Hyperactivity Disorders," in *Introduction to Quantitative EEG and Neurofeedback,* ed. J. R. Evans and A. Abarbanel, 103–143 (New York: Academic Press, 1999).

6. M. A. Sullivan and F. Rudnik-Levin, "Attention Deficit/Hyperactivity Disorder and Substance Abuse: Diagnostic and Therapeutic Considerations," *Annals of the New York Academy of Sciences* 931 (2001): 251–270.

7. S. Donaldson, G. Sella, and H. Mueller, "Fibromyalgia: A Retrospective Study of 252 Consecutive Referrals," *Canadian Journal of Clinical Medicine* 5, no. 6 (1998): 116–127.

8. B. F. Westermoreland, "The EEG in Cerebral Inflamatory Processes," in *Electroencephalography; Basic Principles, Clinical Applications & Related Fields,* ed. E. E. Neidermyer and F. L. DaSilva, vol. 3, 291–304 (Baltimore: Urban Schwartzenberg, 1993).

9. J. Robbins, *A Symphony in the Brain* (New York: Grove Press, 2000), 9.

10. W. Penfield and T. Rasmussen, *The Cerebral Cortex of Man* (New York: Macmillan), 1950.

11. J. Olds, "Pleasure Centres in the Brain," *Scientific American* 195 (1956): 105–116.

12. This study is cited in Robbins, *A Symphony in the Brain,* 23.

13. J. A. Osmundsen, "'Matador' with a Radio Stops Wired Bull," *New York Times,* May 17, 1965, p. 20.

14. L. V. DiCara and N. E. Miller, "Heart-Rate Learning in the Noncurarized State, Transfer to the Curarized State, and Subsequent Retraining in the Noncurarized State," *Physiology and Behavior* 4 (1969): 621–624.

15. Kamiya reported his work on the effects of EEG changes on consciousness in J. Kamiya, "Operant Control of the EEG Alpha Rhythm," in *Altered States of Consciousness, ed.* C. Tart, 507–517 (New York: Wiley, 1969).

16. Joseph LeDoux, professor at New York University's Center for Neural Sciences, provides a fascinating account of the research on the plasticity of "brain circuitry" in *Synaptic Self: How Our Brains Become Who We Are* (New York: Viking, 2002).

17. M. Thompson and L. Thompson, *The Neurofeedback Book: An Introduction to Basic Concepts in Applied Psychophysiology* (Wheat Ridge, Colo.: Association for Applied Psychophysiology and Biofeedback, 2003).

18. J. Cairns, J. Overbaugh, and S. Miller, "The Origin of Mutants," *Nature* 335 (1988): 142–145.

19. M. R. Rosenzweig, "Effects of Differential Experience on the Brain and Behavior," *Developmental Neuropsychology* 24 (2003): 523–540.

20. B. Lipton, *Biology of Belief* (Santa Cruz, Calif.: Elite, 2005).

21. R. W. Thatcher, R. Walker, I. Gerson, and F. Geisler, "EEG Discriminant Analyses of Mild Head Trauma," *Electroencephalography and Clinical Neurophysiology* 73 (1989): 93–106.

22. J. Evans and N. S. Park, "Quantitative EEG Findings among Men Convicted of Murder," *Journal of Neurotheraphy* 2 (1997): 31–39.

23. A good source of information on TBI including prevalence and symptoms is the Brain Injury Association of America website: www.BIAUSA.org.

24. J. van der Naalt, A. H. van Zomeren, W. J. Sluiter, and J. M. Minderhoud, "One Year Outcome in Mild to Moderate Head Injury: The Predictive Value of Acute Injury Characteristics Related to Complaints and Return to Work," *Journal of Neurology, Neurosurgery, and Psychiatry* 66 (1999): 207–213.

25. Thatcher, Walker, Gerson, and Geisler, "EEG Discriminant Analyses of Mild Head Trauma." *Electroencephalography and Clinical Neurophysiology* 73(1989): 93–106.

26. K. Thornton and D. Carmody, "Electroencephalogram Biofeedback for Reading Disability and Traumatic Brain Injury," *Child and Adolescent Psychiatric Clinics of North America* 14 (2005): 137–162.

27. D. A. Hoffman, S. Stockdale, L. L. Hicks, "Diagnosis and Treatment of Head Injury," *Journal of Neurotherapy* 1 (1995): 14–21.

28. J. E. Walker, C. A. Norman, and R. K. Weber, "Impact of QEEG-Guided Coherence Training for Patients with a Mild Closed Head Injury," *Journal of Neurotherapy* 6 (2002): 31–45.

29. A. Byers, "Neurofeedback Therapy for a Mild Head Injury," *Journal of Neurotherapy* 1 (1995): 22–37.

## Chapter 2: How Do Brainwaves Work?

1. R. Shin, "Neuroplasticity in Multiple Sclerosis," *Neurology Reviews* 12 (2004); available online at http://www.neurologyreviews.com/sep04/sep04_nr_neuroplasticityMS.html.

2. A. Amerdi, L. B. Merabet, F. Bermpohl, and A. Pascual-Leone, "The Occipital Cortex in the Blind. Lessons about Plasticity and Vision," *Current Directions in Psychological Science* 14 (2005): 306–311.

3. A. Pascual-Leone and F. Torres, "Plasticity of the Sensorimotor Cortex Representation of the Reading Finger in Braille Readers," *Brain* 116 (1993): 39–52.

4. E. Taub, G. Uswatte, and R. Pidikiti, "Constraint-Induced Movement Therapy: A New Family of Techniques with Broad Application to Physical Rehabilitation—A Clinical Review," *Journal of Rehabilitation Research & Development* 36 (1999); an updated copy is available online at http://www.rehab.research.va.gov/jour/99/36/3/taub.htm.

5. R. W. Thatcher, "EEG Database-Guided Neurotherapy," in *Introduction to Quantitative EEG and Neurofeedback,* ed. J. R. Evans and A. Abarbanel, 29–64 (New York: Academic Press, 1999).

6. E. Green, and A. Green, *Beyond Biofeedback* (Fort Wayne, Ind.: Knoll, 1977).

7. T. Shealy, S. Smith, L. Borgmeyer, and U. Borgmeyer, "EEG Alteration during Absent 'Healing,'" *Subtle Energies and Energy Medicine* 11 (2000): 241–248.

8. D. C. Hammond, "Clinical Hypnosis and Neurofeedback," *Biofeedback* (Spring, 2005): 14–19.

9. M. Doppelmayr, W. Klimesch, W. Stadler, D. Pollhuber, and C. Heine, "Alpha Power and Intelligence," *Intelligence* 30 (2002): 289–302.

10. S. Hanslmayr, P. Sauseng, M. Doppelmayr, M. Schabus, and W. Klimesch, "Increasing Individual Upper Alpha Power by Neurofeedback Improves Cognitive Performance in Human Subjects," *Applied Psychophysiology and Biofeedback* 30 (2005): 1–10.

11. M. Thompson and L. Thompson, *The Neurofeedback Book: An Introduction to Basic Concepts in Applied Psychophysiology* (Wheat Ridge, Colo.: Association for Applied Psychophysiology and Biofeedback, 2003).

12. T. H. Budzynski, "Brain-Brightening," *Biofeedback* (Summer, 1996): 14–17.

13. R. J. Davidson, "Anterior Electrophysiological Asymmetries, Emotion, and Depression: Conceptual and Methodological Conundrums," *Psychophysiology* 35 (1998): 607–614.

14. W. Wyrwicka and M. B. Sterman, "Instrumental Conditioning of Sensorimotor Cortex EEG Spindles in the Waking Cat," *Physiology and Behavior* 3 (1968): 703–707.

15. An excellent account of Sterman's discovery of the effects of SMR training on seizure threshold can be found in Jim Robbins's *A Symphony in the Brain* (New York: Grove Press, 2000), 32–43.

16. Ibid., 32–52.

17. P. G. Swingle, "Neurofeedback Treatment of Pseudoseizure Disorder," *Biological Psychiatry* 44 (1998): 1196–1199.

18. L. B. Holmes, E. A. Harvey, B. A. Coull, K. B. Huntington, S. Khoshbin, A. M. Hayes, and L. M. Ryan, "The Teratogenicity of Anticonvulsant Drugs," *New England Journal of Medicine* 344 (2001): 1132–1138.

19. M. B. Sterman, "Basic Concepts and Clinical Findings in the Treatment of Seizure Disorders with EEG Operant Conditioning," *Clinical Electroencephalography* 31 (2000): 45–54.

20. D. A. Quirk, "Composite Biofeedback Conditioning and Dangerous Offenders: III," *Journal of Neurotherapy* 1(1995): 44–54.

21. J. S. Kim, S. Choi, S. Kwon, and Y. S. Seo, "Inability to Control Anger or Aggression after Stroke," *Neurology* 58 (2002): 1106–1108.

22. A. Strohmayer, "SMR Neurofeedback Efficacy in the Treatment of Tourette Syndrome" (paper presented at the meetings of the International Society for Neuronal Regulation, Ft. Lauderdale, Fla., 2004).

23. R. Daly and B. Lev, "Tourette's Syndrome: Three-Year Follow-up of a Successful Treatment Outcome" (paper presented at the meetings of the International Society for Neuronal Regulation, Houston, 2003).

24. D. C. Hammond, "Neurofeedback with Anxiety and Affective Disorders," *Child and Adolescent Psychiatric Clinics of North America* 14 (2005): 105–123.

25. P. G. Swingle, "Potentiating Neurotherapy: Techniques for Stimulating the EEG," *California Biofeedback* (Summer, 2003).

## Chapter 3: Interpreting the Signals of the Brain

1. M. A. Schuckit, T. L. Smith, J. Kalmijn, J. Tsuang, V. Hesselbrock, and K. Bucholz, "Response to Alcohol in Daughters of Alcoholics: A Pilot Study and a Comparsion with Sons of Alcoholics," *Alcohol and Alcoholism* 35 (2000): 242–248.

2. D. L. Thombs, "Introduction," *Addictive Behaviors,* 3rd ed. (New York: Guilford Press, 2006).

3. J. R. Hughes and E. R. John, "Conventional and Quantitative Electroencephalography in Psychiatry," *Journal of Neuropsychiatry and Clinical Neurosciences* 11 (1999): 190–208.

4. B. Simpson, "Symptom Provocation Alters Behavioural Ratings and Brain Electrical Activity in Obsessive-Compulsive Disorder: A Preliminary Study," *Psychiatry Research* 95 (2000): 149–155.

5. H. Ashton, "The Treatment of Benzodiazepine Dependence," *Addiction* 89 (1994): 1535–1541.

6. L. Thompson and M. Thompson, *The Neurofeedback Book: An Introduction to Basic Concepts in Applied Psychophysiology* (Wheat Ridge, Colo.: Association for Applied Psychophysiology and Biofeedback, 2003).

7. M. B. Stein, K. L. Jang, S. Taylor, P. A. Vernon, and W. J. Livesley, "Genetic and Environmental Influences on Trauma Exposure and Posttraumatic Stress Disorder Symptoms: A Twin Study," *American Journal of Psychiatry* 159 (2002): 1675–1681.

8. L. S. Prichep, S. C. Kowalik, K. Alper, and C. deJesus, "Quantitative EEG Characteristics of Children Exposed in Utero to Cocaine," *Clinical Electroencephalography* 26 (1995): 166–172.

9. C. J. Brainerd and V. F. Reyna, *The Science of False Memory* (New York: Oxford University Press, 2005).

10. T. P. Sbraga and W. O'Donohue, "Post Hoc Reasoning in Possible Cases of Child Sexual Abuse: Symptoms of Inconclusive Origins," *Clinical Psychology: Science and Practice* 10 (2003): 320–334.

11. M. Doppelmayr, W. Klimesch, W. Stadler, D. Pollhuber, and C. Heine, "Alpha Power and Intelligence," *Intelligence* 30 (2002): 289–302.

12. Thompson and Thompson, *The Neurofeedback Book, 225.*

13. S. M. Suldo, A. Olson, and J. R. Evans, "Quantitative EEG Evidence of Increased Alpha Peak Frequency in Children with Precocious Reading Ability," *Journal of Neurotherapy* 5 (2001): 39–50.

14. R. Weinstein, "QEEG in Death Penalty Evaluations" (paper presented at the meeting of the International Society for Neuronal Regulation, Phoenix, 2002).

15. R. J. Davidson, "Cerebral Asymmetry, Emotion and Affective Style." In *Brain Asymmetry,* ed. R. J. Davidson and K. Hugdahl, 369–388 (Cambridge, Mass.: MIT Press, 1995).

## Chapter 4: Neurotherapy and Its Partners in Treatment

1. N. Lindberg, P. Tani, M. Virkkunen, T. Porkka-Heiskanen, B. Appelberg, H. Naukkarinen, and T. Salmi, "Quantitative Electroencephalographic Measures in Homicidal Men with Antisocial Personality Disorder," *Psychiatry Research* 136 (2005): 7–15.

2. National Institutes of Health, *Consensus Statement "Diagnosis and Treatment of ADHD,"* 1998, available online at www.NIH.gov.

3. J. H. Satterfield and A. Norman, "Response to Stimulant Drug Treatment in Hyperactive Children," *Annals of the New York Academy of Sciences* 205 (1973): 274–282.

4. J. F. Lubar, and J. O. Lubar, "Neurofeedback Assessment and Treatment for Attention Deficit/Hyperactivity Disorders," in *Introduction to Quantitative EEG and Neurofeedback,* ed. J. R. Evans and A. Abarbanel, 103–143 (New York: Academic Press, 1999).

5. B. P. Mruz, D. D. Montgomery, W. J. Burns, K. A. Owen, A. C. Chang, and A. Braten, "Effects of AVS Dominant Frequency Disentrainment on QEEG in a Sample of Normal Adults" (paper presented at the annual meeting of the Association for Applied Psychophysiology and Biofeedback, March 2003, Jacksonville, Fla.); abstract in *Applied Psychophysiology and Biofeedback* 28 (2003): 315–316.

6. The 1995 and 1998 research as well as abstracts of other research on the benefits of CES can be found in D. L. Kirsch, *The Science Behind Cranial Electrical Stimulation,* 2nd ed. (Edmonton, Alberta: Medical Scope Publishing, 2002).

7. R. Smith, "Is Microcurrent Stimulation Effective in Pain Management? An Additional Perspective," *Journal of Pain Management* 11, no. 2 (2001): 62–66.

8. R. Kennerly, "QEEG Analysis of Cranial Electrotherapy: A Pilot Study (Abstract)," *Journal of Neurotherapy* 8 (2004): 112–113; presented at the International Society for Neuronal Regulation annual conference, Sept. 18–21, 2003, Houston.

9. C. L. Zhang, "Skin Resistance vs. Body Conductivity: On the Background of Electronic Measurement on Skin," *Subtle Energies & Energy Medicine* 14 (2003): 151–174.

10. P. G. Swingle, L. Pulos, and M. Swingle, "Neurophysiological Indicators of EFT Treatment of Post-Traumatic Stress," *Subtle Energies & Energy Medicine* 15 (2003): 75–86.

11. P. G. Swingle, "Emotional Freedom Technique (EFT) and Theta Suppressing Harmonic Markedly Accelerates SMR Treatment of Seizure Disorders" (paper presented at the meeting of the Association for Applied Psychophysiology and Biofeedback, Raleigh, N.C., March 2001).

12. P. G. Swingle, "Neurofeedback Treatment of Pseudoseizure Disorder," *Biological Psychiatry* 44 (1998): 1196–1199.

13. Glen's real name is Adam, and his courageous mother, Arlene, has written a helpful book about her experiences getting adequate treatment for her son's seizure disorder and autism. The book is available on the web at: www.gettingadamback.com. Arlene wrote to me on May 7, 2007, with an update: "After treatments, Adam's obsessive compulsive behaviour is almost nonexistent. He was able to come off the Ketogenic diet and today is seizure free, drug free and 90% of his autistic tendencies are gone. He functions at a level that I would have only dreamed of previously. He is extremely sociable, friendly and well liked by his peers. He is well mannered and has a really positive outlook on life. Although he still needs some reminders when it comes to life skills, he does most everything on his own and continues to work on his independence."

14. P. G. Swingle, "Subthreshold 10Hz Sound Suppresses EEG Theta: Clinical Application for the Potentiation of Neurotherapeutic Treatment of ADD/ADHD," *Journal of Neurotherapy* 2 (1996): 15–22.

15. B. L. Gruber and E. Taub, "Thermal and EMG Biofeedback Learning in Nonhuman Primates," *Applied Psychophysiology and Biofeedback* 23 (1998): 1–12.

16. W. Boyd and S. Campbell, "EEG Biofeedback in the Schools: The Use of EEG Biofeedback to Treat ADHD in a School Setting," *Journal of Neurotherapy* 2 (1998): 65–70.

17. D. Carmody, D. Radvanski, S. Wadhwani, J. Sabo, and L. Vergara, "EEG Biofeedback Training and Attention-Deficit/Hyperactivity Disorder in an Elementary School Setting," *Journal of Neurotherapy* 4 (2001): 5–27.

## Chapter 5: Diagnostic Chaos: The Case of ADHD

1. F. J. Zimmerman, G. M. Glew, D. A. Christakis, and W. Katon, "Early Cognitive Stimulation, Emotional Support, and Television Watching as Predictors of Subsequent Bullying among Grade-School Children," *Archives of Pediatric Adolescent Medicine* 159 (2005): 384–388.

2. P. Rodkin and E. Hodges, "Bullies and Victims in the Peer Ecology: Four Questions for Psychologists and School Professionals," *School Psychology Review* 32 (2003): 382–400.

3. D. L. Espelage and S. M. Swearer, "Research on School Bullying and Victimization: What Have We Learned and Where Do We Go from Here?" *School Psychology Review* 32 (2003): 365–383.

4. Further helpful information can be found on the website of the American Academy of Pediatrics: www.AAP.org.

5. S. V. Faraone, J. Biederman, E. Mick, S. Williamson, T. Wilens, T. Spencer, W. Weber, J. Jetton, I. Kraus, J. Pert, and B. Zallen, "Family Study of Girls with Attention Deficit Hyperactivity Disorder," *American Journal of Psychiatry* 157 (2000): 1077–1083.

6. R. D. Hunt, "An Update on Assessment and Treatment of Complex Attention-Deficit/Hyperactivity Disorder," *Pediatric Annals* 30 (2001): 163.

7. F. Levy and D. A. Hay, *Attention Genes and ADHD* (Hove, East Sussex: Taylor and Francis; Philadelphia: Brunner-Routledge, 2001).

8. G. Maté, *Scattered Minds* (Toronto: Vintage Canada, 2000).

9. T. Hartman, *Attention Deficit Disorder: A Different Perspective* (Nevada City, Calif.: Underwood Books, 1997).

10. P. Quinn and S. Wigal, "Perceptions of Girls and ADHD: Results from a National Survey," *Medscape: General Medicine,* http://www.medscape.com/viewarticle/472415, posted May 4, 2004.

11. A. Gutman and J. Spollen, "ADHD Perspectives from Child to Adult" (paper presented at the meeting of the American Association of Child and Adolescent Psychiatry, San Francisco, October 2002).

12. L. Adler, D. J. Sitt, A. Nierenberg, and H. D. Mandler, "Patterns of Psychiatric Comorbidity with Attention Deficit Hyperactivity Disorder" (paper presented at the 19th U.S. Psychiatric & Mental Health Congress, November 15–19, 2006, New Orleans, Abstract 119).

13. J. J. McGough, S. L. Smalley, J. T. McCracken, M. Yang, M. Del'Homme, D. E. Lynn, and S. Loo, "Psychiatric Comorbidity in Adult Attention Deficit Hyperactivity Disorder: Findings from Multiplex Families," *American Journal of Psychiatry* 162 (2005): 1621–1627.

14. Quinn and Wigal, "Perceptions of Girls and ADHD."

15. H. Elliot, "Attention Deficit Hyperactivity Disorder in Adults: A Guide for the Primary Care Physician," *Southern Medical Journal* 95 (2002): 736–742.

16. P. G. Swingle, "Potentiating Neurotherapy: Techniques for Stimulating the EEG," *California Biofeedback* (Summer, 2003).

17. P. G. Swingle, "Parameters Associated with Rapid Neurotherapeutic Treatment of Common ADD (CADD)," *Journal of Neurotherapy* 5 (2001): 73–84.

18. P. G. Swingle, "The Practice of Neurotherapy," unpublished manuscript.

19. J. Thomas and B. Sattlberger, "Treatment of Chronic Anxiety Disorder with Neurotherapy: A Case Study," *Journal of Neurotherapy* 2 (1997): 14–19.

20. M. Johann, G. Bobbe, A. Putzhammer, and N. Wodarz, "Comorbidity of Alcohol Dependence with Attention-Deficit Hyperactivity Disorder: Differences in Phenotype with Increased Severity of the Substance Disorder, but Not in Genotype (Serotonin Transporter and 5-Hydroxytryptamine-2c Receptor)," *Alcoholism: Clinical & Experimental Research* 27(2003): 1527–1534; K. Tasmussen, R. Almvik, and S. Levander, "Attention Deficit Disorder, Reading Disability, and Personality Disorders in a Prison Population," *Journal of the American Academy of Psychiatry and the Law* 29 (2001): 186–193.

21. S. Goldstein, "Attention-Deficit/Hyperactivity Disorder: Implications for the Criminal Justice System," *FBI Law Enforcement Bulletin* (June 1997). Goldstein's review article citing these and related statistics is available on the FBI publications website: http://www.fbi.gov/publications/leb/1997/june973.htm.

22. M. A. Sullivan and F. Rudnik-Levin, "Attention Deficit/Hyperactivity Disorder and Substance Abuse: Diagnostic and Therapeutic Considerations," *Annals of the New York Academy of Sciences* 931 (2001): 251–270.

23. R. J. Davidson, and K. Hugdahl, eds., *Brain Asymmetry* (Cambridge, Mass.: MIT Press, 1995).

24. E. Baehr, J. Rosenfeld, and R. Baehr, "Clinical Use of an Alpha Asymmetry Neurofeedback Protocol in the Treatment of Mood Disorders: Follow-Up Study One to Five Years post Therapy," *Journal of Neurotherapy* 4 (2001): 11–18.

25. R. Weinstein, "QEEG in Death Penalty Evaluations" (paper presented at the meeting of the International Society for Neuronal Regulation, Phoenix, 2002).

## Chapter 6: The Broad Reach of Neurotherapy

1. W. A. Carlezon Jr. and C. Konradi, "Understanding the Neurobiological Consequences of Early Exposure to Psychotropic Drugs: Linking Behavior with Molecules," *Neuropharmacology* 47S1 (2004): 47–60.

2. S. Shea, A. Turgay, A. Carroll, M. Schulz, H. Orlik, I. Smith, and F. Dunbar, "Risperidone in the Treatment of Disruptive Behavioral Symptoms in Children with Autistic and Other Pervasive Developmental Disorders," *Pediatrics* 114 (2004): 634–641.

3. P. Whybrow, *American Mania* (New York: Norton, 2005); P. Whybrow, *A Mood Apart* (New York: HarperCollins, 1997). The quote is from "Mood Disorders at the Turn of the Century: An Expert Interview with Peter C. Whybrow, MD," *Medscape Psychiatry & Mental Health,* http://www.medscape.com/viewarticle/503013, posted May 19, 2005.

4. J. Walker, C. Norman, and R. Weber, "Impact of QEEG-Guided Coherence Training for Patients with a Mild Closed Head Injury," *Journal of Neurotherapy* 6 (2002): 31–43.

5. T. Tinius, *New Developments in Blood Flow Hemoencephalography* (Binghamton, N.Y.: Haworth Press, 2004).

6. E. Fombonne, "Epidemiological Surveys of Autism and Other Pervasive Developmental Disorders," *Journal of Autism and Developmental Disorders* 33 (2003): 365–382.

7. S. Klein and J. Kilstrom, "On Bridging the Gap between Social-Personality Psychology and Neuropsychology," *Personality and Social Psychology Review* 2 (1998): 228–242.

8. E. R. Braverman and K. Blum, "Substance Use Disorder Exacerbates Brain Electrophysiological Abnormalities in a Psychiatrically Ill Population," *Clinical Electroencephalography* 27a (1996): 5–28.

9. M. S. Scher, G. A. Richardson, and N. L. Day, "Effects of Prenatal Cocaine/Crack and Other Drug Exposure on Electroencephalographic Sleep Studies at Birth and One Year," *Pediatrics* 105 (2000): 39–48.

10. C. Chiriboga, "Fetal Alcohol and Drug Effects," *Neurologist* 9 (2003): 267–279.

11. R. Hill and E. Castro, *Getting Rid of Ritalin* (Charlottesville, Vir.: Hampton Roads, 2002).

12. R. Barkley, *Attention Deficit Hyperactivity Disorder: A Handbook for Diagnosis and Treatment*, 3rd ed. (New York: Guilford, 2006).

13. National Institutes of Health, *Consensus Statement "Diagnosis and Treatment of ADHD,"* 1998, available online at www.NIH.gov.

14. S. Goldstein and M. Goldstein, *Managing Attention Disorders in Children: A Guide for Practitioners* (New York: Wiley, 1990).

15. L. L. Greenhill, J. M. Halperin, and H. Abikoff, "Stimulant Medication," *Journal of the American Academy of Child and Adolescent Psychiatry* 38 (1999): 503–512.

16. P. Breggin, *Talking Back to Ritalin, Revised :What Doctors Aren't Telling You about Stimulants and ADHD* (New York: Perseus Books, 2001).

17. N. D. Volkow, G. J. Wang, J. S. Fowler, J. Logan, M. Gerasimov, L. Maynard, Y. S. Ding, S. J. Gatley, A. Gifford, and D. Franceschi, "Therapeutic Doses of Oral Methylphenidate Significantly Increase Extracellular Dopamine in the Human Brain," *Journal of Neuroscience* 21 (2001): 1–5.

18. S. E. McCabe, C. J. Teter, and C. J. Boyd, "The Use, Misuse and Diversion of Prescription Stimulants among Middle and High School Students," *Substance Use Misuse* 39 (2004): 1095–1116.

19. B. P. White, K. A. Becker-Blease, and K. Grace-Bishop, "Stimulant Medication Use, Misuse, and Abuse in an Undergraduate and Graduate Student Sample," *Journal of American College Health* 54 (2006): 261–268.

20. T. Wilens, "Diversion and Misuse of Stimulant ADHD Medications Uncommon in the Absence of Comorbid Disorders" (paper presented at the American Psychiatric Association annual meeting, 2005, Abstract 9).

21. J. M. Zito, D. J. Safer, S. dosReis, J. F. Gardner, M. Boles, and F. Lynch, "Trends in the Prescribing of Psychotropic Medications to Preschoolers," *Journal of the American Medical Association* 283 (2000): 1025–1030.

22. Lawrence Diller, author of *The Last Normal Child* (New York: Praeger, 2006), stated in "Don't Drug Them," *San Francisco Chronicle,* Nov. 19, 2006, that one medical-insurance clearinghouse reported that about one in ten white, eleven-year-old male children was on a stimulant medication. He further stated that the use of stimulant medication in children had grown by about 2000 percent in the previous fifteen years. A study reported by the American Society of Health System Pharmacists (available on-line at www.safemedication.com) found that nearly three fourths (72.8 percent) of households have at least one person taking a prescription medication and in nearly half (47.6 percent) one person is taking three or more prescription medications. A sample of 1.9 million life-years of commercially insured children age eighteen years and under in the United States showed that between 1998 and 2002 prescriptions for antidepressant medications increased 9.4 percent annually; in 2002, 2.4 percent of all children surveyed were taking antidepressant medications, and the highest use was by fifteen- to eighteen-year-old females, of whom 6.4 percent were on antidepressants (T. Delate, A. J. Gelenberg, V. A. Simmons, and B. R. Motheral, "Trends in the Use of Antidepressants in a National Sample of Commercially Insured Pediatric Patients, 1998 to 2002," *Psychiatric Services* 55 (2004): 387–391). In 2001, one out of ten office visits by adolescent males in the United States resulted in a prescription for a psychotropic medication according to the National Ambulatory Medical Care Survey, reported in C. P. Thomas, P. Conrad,

R. Casler, and E. Goodman, "Trends in the Use of Psychotropic Medications among Adolescents, 1994 to 2001," *Psychiatric Services* 57 (2006): 79–83. The number of children prescribed antipsychotic drugs annually jumped almost fivefold between 1995 and 2002; in the mid-1990s, 8.6 out of every 1,000 children were prescribed antipsychotic medications whereas in 2002 it was nearly 40 out of 1,000 (W. Cooper, P. Arbogast, H. Ding, G. Hickson, D. Fuchs, and W. Ray, "Trends in Prescribing of Antipsychotic Medications for US Children," *Ambulatory Pediatrics* 6 (2006): 63–69).

23. Quote is from P. Breggin's website, http://www.breggin.com/ritalinexcerpt.html, which contains summaries and excerpts from his book *Talking Back to Ritalin* (see note 16 above).

24. A. Tonkin and J. Jureidini, "Wishful Thinking: Antidepressant Drugs in Childhood Depression," *British Journal of Psychiatry* 187 (2005): 304–305.

25. Details of the relationship between inadequate development of the ROFC and psychophysiological disorders can be found in A. Schore, *Affect Dysregulation and Disorders of the Self* (New York: Norton, 2003).

26. J. P. Murray, "TV Violence and Brainmapping in Children," *Psychiatric Times* 18 (2001): 70–71.

27. The guidelines and recommendations of the American Academy of Pediatrics are available on the Academy's website: www.aap.org/family/mediaimpact.htm.

28. J. Funk, H. Baldacci, T. Pasold, and J. Baumgardner, "Violence Exposure in Real Life, Video Games, Television, Movies and the Internet. Is There Desensitization?" *Journal of Adolescence* 27 (2004): 23–39.

29. D. Gentile, P. Lynch, J. Linder, and D. Walsh, "The Effects of Violent Video Game Habits on Adolescent Hostility, Aggressive Behaviors, and School Performance," *Journal of Adolescence* 27 (2004): 5–22.

## Chapter 7: The Promise of Neurotherapy in the Future

1. A complete discussion of LORETA and the relevant research can be found at http://www.unizh.ch/keyinst/NewLORETA/LORETA01.htm#WhatIsLORETA.

# INDEX

## ABOUT THE AUTHOR

Paul G. Swingle was professor of psychology at the University of Ottawa from 1972 to 1997; he was chair of the faculty of child psychology there from 1972 to 1977 and a clinical supervisor from 1987 to 1997. A fellow of the Canadian Psychological Association, Dr. Swingle was lecturer in psychiatry at Harvard Medical School from 1991 to 1998 and during the same time period was associate attending psychologist at McLean Hospital (Boston), where he also was coordinator of the Clinical Psychophysiology Service. He currently lives in Vancouver, British Columbia, where he is a registered psychologist and is certified in biofeedback and neurotherapy.